**Mental Health Policy and
Service Guidance Package**

MENTAL HEALTH
LEGISLATION &
HUMAN RIGHTS

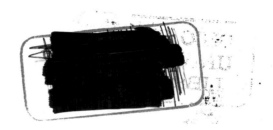

World Health Organization, 2003

WHO Library Cataloguing-in-Publication Data

Mental health legislation and human rights.
(Mental health policy and service guidance package)

1. Mental health - legislation
2. Patient rights - legislation
3. Mentally ill persons - legislation
4. Health policy
5. National health programs - legislation
6. Guidelines   I. World Health Organization   II. Series.

ISBN 92 4 154595 x
(NLM classification: WM 30)

Technical information concerning this publication can be obtained from:
Dr Michelle Funk
Mental Health Policy and Service Development Team
Department of Mental Health and Substance Dependence
Noncommunicable Diseases and Mental Health Cluster
World Health Organization
CH-1211, Geneva 27
Switzerland
Tel: +41 22 791 3855
Fax: +41 22 791 4160
E-mail: funkm@who.int

Printed in Singapore.

Acknowledgements

The Mental Health Policy and Service Guidance Package was produced under the direction of Dr Michelle Funk, Coordinator, Mental Health Policy and Service Development, and supervised by Dr Benedetto Saraceno, Director, Department of Mental Health and Substance Dependence, World Health Organization.

The World Health Organization gratefully acknowledges the work of Dr Soumitra Pathare, Ruby Hall Clinic, Pune, India and Dr Alberto Minoletti, Ministry of Health, Chile, who prepared this module.

Editorial and technical coordination group:

Dr Michelle Funk, World Health Organization, Headquarters (WHO/HQ), Ms Natalie Drew, (WHO/HQ), Dr JoAnne Epping-Jordan, (WHO/HQ), Professor Alan J. Flisher, University of Cape Town, Observatory, Republic of South Africa, Professor Melvyn Freeman, Department of Health, Pretoria, South Africa, Dr Howard Goldman, National Association of State Mental Health Program Directors Research Institute and University of Maryland School of Medicine, USA, Dr Itzhak Levav, Mental Health Services, Ministry of Health, Jerusalem, Israel and Dr Benedetto Saraceno, (WHO/HQ).

Dr Crick Lund, University of Cape Town, Observatory, Republic of South Africa, finalized the technical editing of this module.

Technical assistance:

Dr Jose Bertolote, World Health Organization, Headquarters (WHO/HQ), Dr Thomas Bornemann (WHO/HQ), Dr José Miguel Caldas de Almeida, WHO Regional Office for the Americas (AMRO), Dr Vijay Chandra, WHO Regional Office for South-East Asia (SEARO), Dr Custodia Mandlhate, WHO Regional Office for Africa (AFRO), Dr Claudio Miranda (AMRO), Dr Ahmed Mohit, WHO Regional Office for the Eastern Mediterranean, Dr Wolfgang Rutz, WHO Regional Office for Europe (EURO), Dr Erica Wheeler (WHO/HQ), Dr Derek Yach (WHO/HQ), and staff of the WHO Evidence and Information for Policy Cluster (WHO/HQ).

Administrative and secretarial support:

Ms Adeline Loo (WHO/HQ), Mrs Anne Yamada (WHO/HQ) and Mrs Razia Yaseen (WHO/HQ).

Layout and graphic design: 2S) graphicdesign
Editor: Walter Ryder

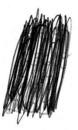

WHO also gratefully thanks the following people for their expert opinion and technical input to this module:

Dr Adel Hamid Afana	Director, Training and Education Department Gaza Community Mental Health Programme
Dr Bassam Al Ashhab	Ministry of Health, Palestinian Authority, West Bank
Mrs Ella Amir	Ami Québec, Canada
Dr Julio Arboleda-Florez	Department of Psychiatry, Queen's University, Kingston, Ontario, Canada
Ms Jeannine Auger	Ministry of Health and Social Services, Québec, Canada
Dr Florence Baingana	World Bank, Washington DC, USA
Mrs Louise Blanchette	University of Montreal Certificate Programme in Mental Health, Montreal, Canada
Dr Susan Blyth	University of Cape Town, Cape Town, South Africa
Ms Nancy Breitenbach	Inclusion International, Ferney-Voltaire, France
Dr Anh Thu Bui	Ministry of Health, Koror, Republic of Palau
Dr Sylvia Caras	People Who Organization, Santa Cruz, California, USA
Dr Claudina Cayetano	Ministry of Health, Belmopan, Belize
Dr Chueh Chang	Taipei, Taiwan
Professor Yan Fang Chen	Shandong Mental Health Centre, Jinan People's Republic of China
Dr Chantharavdy Choulamany	Mahosot General Hospital, Vientiane, Lao People's Democratic Republic
Dr Ellen Corin	Douglas Hospital Research Centre, Quebec, Canada
Dr Jim Crowe	President, World Fellowship for Schizophrenia and Allied Disorders, Dunedin, New Zealand
Dr Araba Sefa Dedeh	University of Ghana Medical School, Accra, Ghana
Dr Nimesh Desai	Professor of Psychiatry and Medical Superintendent, Institute of Human Behaviour and Allied Sciences, India
Dr M. Parameshvara Deva	Department of Psychiatry, Perak College of Medicine, Ipoh, Perak, Malaysia
Professor Saida Douki	President, Société Tunisienne de Psychiatrie, Tunis, Tunisia
Professor Ahmed Abou El-Azayem	Past President, World Federation for Mental Health, Cairo, Egypt
Dr Abra Fransch	WONCA, Harare, Zimbabwe
Dr Gregory Fricchione	Carter Center, Atlanta, USA
Dr Michael Friedman	Nathan S. Kline Institute for Psychiatric Research, Orangeburg, NY, USA
Mrs Diane Froggatt	Executive Director, World Fellowship for Schizophrenia and Allied Disorders, Toronto, Ontario, Canada
Mr Gary Furlong	Metro Local Community Health Centre, Montreal, Canada
Dr Vijay Ganju	National Association of State Mental Health Program Directors Research Institute, Alexandria, VA, USA
Mrs Reine Gobeil	Douglas Hospital, Quebec, Canada
Dr Nacanieli Goneyali	Ministry of Health, Suva, Fiji
Dr Gaston Harnois	Douglas Hospital Research Centre, WHO Collaborating Centre, Quebec, Canada
Mr Gary Haugland	Nathan S. Kline Institute for Psychiatric Research, Orangeburg, NY, USA
Dr Yanling He	Consultant, Ministry of Health, Beijing, People's Republic of China
Professor Helen Herrman	Department of Psychiatry, University of Melbourne, Australia

Mrs Karen Hetherington	WHO/PAHO Collaborating Centre, Canada
Professor Frederick Hickling	Section of Psychiatry, University of West Indies, Kingston, Jamaica
Dr Kim Hopper	Nathan S. Kline Institute for Psychiatric Research, Orangeburg, NY, USA
Dr Tae-Yeon Hwang	Director, Department of Psychiatric Rehabilitation and Community Psychiatry, Yongin City, Republic of Korea
Dr A. Janca	University of Western Australia, Perth, Australia
Dr Dale L. Johnson	World Fellowship for Schizophrenia and Allied Disorders, Taos, NM, USA
Dr Kristine Jones	Nathan S. Kline Institute for Psychiatric Research, Orangeburg, NY, USA
Dr David Musau Kiima	Director, Department of Mental Health, Ministry of Health, Nairobi, Kenya
Mr Todd Krieble	Ministry of Health, Wellington, New Zealand
Mr John P. Kummer	Equilibrium, Unteraegeri, Switzerland
Professor Lourdes Ladrido-Ignacio	Department of Psychiatry and Behavioural Medicine, College of Medicine and Philippine General Hospital, Manila, Philippines
Dr Pirkko Lahti	Secretary-General/Chief Executive Officer, World Federation for Mental Health, and Executive Director, Finnish Association for Mental Health, Helsinki, Finland
Mr Eero Lahtinen,	Ministry of Social Affairs and Health, Helsinki, Finland
Dr Eugene M. Laska	Nathan S. Kline Institute for Psychiatric Research, Orangeburg, NY, USA
Dr Eric Latimer	Douglas Hospital Research Centre, Quebec, Canada
Dr Ian Lockhart	University of Cape Town, Observatory, Republic of South Africa
Dr Marcelino López	Research and Evaluation, Andalusian Foundation for Social Integration of the Mentally Ill, Seville, Spain
Ms Annabel Lyman	Behavioural Health Division, Ministry of Health, Koror, Republic of Palau
Dr Ma Hong	Consultant, Ministry of Health, Beijing, People's Republic of China
Dr George Mahy	University of the West Indies, St Michael, Barbados
Dr Joseph Mbatia	Ministry of Health, Dar-es-Salaam, Tanzania
Dr Céline Mercier	Douglas Hospital Research Centre, Quebec, Canada
Dr Leen Meulenbergs	Belgian Inter-University Centre for Research and Action, Health and Psychobiological and Psychosocial Factors, Brussels, Belgium
Dr Harry I. Minas	Centre for International Mental Health and Transcultural Psychiatry, St. Vincent's Hospital, Fitzroy, Victoria, Australia
Dr Alberto Minoletti	Ministry of Health, Santiago de Chile, Chile
Dr P. Mogne	Ministry of Health, Mozambique
Dr Paul Morgan	SANE, South Melbourne, Victoria, Australia
Dr Driss Moussaoui	Université psychiatrique, Casablanca, Morocco
Dr Matt Muijen	The Sainsbury Centre for Mental Health, London, United Kingdom
Dr Carmine Munizza	Centro Studi e Ricerca in Psichiatria, Turin, Italy
Dr Shisram Narayan	St Giles Hospital, Suva, Fiji
Dr Sheila Ndyanabangi	Ministry of Health, Kampala, Uganda
Dr Grayson Norquist	National Institute of Mental Health, Bethesda, MD, USA
Dr Frank Njenga	Chairman of Kenya Psychiatrists' Association, Nairobi, Kenya

Dr Angela Ofori-Atta	Clinical Psychology Unit, University of Ghana Medical School, Korle-Bu, Ghana
Professor Mehdi Paes	Arrazi University Psychiatric Hospital, Sale, Morocco
Dr Rampersad Parasram	Ministry of Health, Port of Spain, Trinidad and Tobago
Dr Vikram Patel	Sangath Centre, Goa, India
Dr Dixianne Penney	Nathan S. Kline Institute for Psychiatric Research, Orangeburg, NY, USA
Dr Yogan Pillay	Equity Project, Pretoria, Republic of South Africa
Dr M. Pohanka	Ministry of Health, Czech Republic
Dr Laura L. Post	Mariana Psychiatric Services, Saipan, USA
Dr Prema Ramachandran	Planning Commission, New Delhi, India
Dr Helmut Remschmidt	Department of Child and Adolescent Psychiatry, Marburg, Germany
Professor Brian Robertson	Department of Psychiatry, University of Cape Town, Republic of South Africa
Dr Julieta Rodriguez Rojas	Integrar a la Adolescencia, Costa Rica
Dr Agnes E. Rupp	Chief, Mental Health Economics Research Program, NIMH/NIH, USA
Dr Ayesh M. Sammour	Ministry of Health, Palestinian Authority, Gaza
Dr Aive Sarjas	Department of Social Welfare, Tallinn, Estonia
Dr Radha Shankar	AASHA (Hope), Chennai, India
Dr Carole Siegel	Nathan S. Kline Institute for Psychiatric Research, Orangeburg, NY, USA
Professor Michele Tansella	Department of Medicine and Public Health, University of Verona, Italy
Ms Mrinali Thalgodapitiya	Executive Director, NEST, Hendala, Watala, Gampaha District, Sri Lanka
Dr Graham Thornicroft	Director, PRISM, The Maudsley Institute of Psychiatry, London, United Kingdom
Dr Giuseppe Tibaldi	Centro Studi e Ricerca in Psichiatria, Turin, Italy
Ms Clare Townsend	Department of Psychiatry, University of Queensland, Toowing Qld, Australia
Dr Gombodorjiin Tsetsegdary	Ministry of Health and Social Welfare, Mongolia
Dr Bogdana Tudorache	President, Romanian League for Mental Health, Bucharest, Romania
Ms Judy Turner-Crowson	Former Chair, World Association for Psychosocial Rehabilitation, WAPR Advocacy Committee, Hamburg, Germany
Mrs Pascale Van den Heede	Mental Health Europe, Brussels, Belgium
Ms Marianna Várfalvi-Bognarne	Ministry of Health, Hungary
Dr Uldis Veits	Riga Municipal Health Commission, Riga, Latvia
Mr Luc Vigneault	Association des Groupes de Défense des Droits en Santé Mentale du Québec, Canada
Dr Liwei Wang	Consultant, Ministry of Health, Beijing, People's Republic of China
Dr Xiangdong Wang	Acting Regional Adviser for Mental Health, WHO Regional Office for the Western Pacific, Manila, Philippines
Professor Harvey Whiteford	Department of Psychiatry, University of Queensland, Toowing Qld, Australia
Dr Ray G. Xerri	Department of Health, Floriana, Malta
Dr Xie Bin	Consultant, Ministry of Health, Beijing, People's Republic of China
Dr Xin Yu	Consultant, Ministry of Health, Beijing, People's Republic of China
Professor Shen Yucun	Institute of Mental Health, Beijing Medical University, People's Republic of China

Dr Taintor Zebulon   President, WAPR, Department of Psychiatry,
                               New York University Medical Center, New York, USA

WHO also wishes to acknowledge the generous financial support of the Governments of Australia, Finland, Italy, the Netherlands, New Zealand, and Norway, as well as the Eli Lilly and Company Foundation and the Johnson and Johnson Corporate Social Responsibility, Europe.

"All people with mental disorders have the right to receive high quality treatment and care delivered through responsive health care services. They should be protected against any form of inhuman treatment and discrimination."

Table of Contents

This module is part of the WHO Mental Health Policy and Service guidance package, which provides practical information to assist countries to improve the mental health of their populations.

What is the purpose of the guidance package?

The purpose of the guidance package is to assist policy-makers and planners to:

- develop policies and comprehensive strategies for improving the mental health of populations;

- use existing resources to achieve the greatest possible benefits;

- provide effective services to those in need;

- assist the reintegration of persons with mental disorders into all aspects of community life, thus improving their overall quality of life.

What is in the package?

The package consists of a series of interrelated user-friendly modules that are designed to address the wide variety of needs and priorities in policy development and service planning. The topic of each module represents a core aspect of mental health. The starting point is the module entitled The Mental Health Context, which outlines the global context of mental health and summarizes the content of all the modules. This module should give readers an understanding of the global context of mental health, and should enable them to select specific modules that will be useful to them in their own situations. Mental Health Policy, Plans and Programmes is a central module, providing detailed information about the process of developing policy and implementing it through plans and programmes. Following a reading of this module, countries may wish to focus on specific aspects of mental health covered in other modules.

The guidance package includes the following modules:

> The Mental Health Context
> Mental Health Policy, Plans and Programmes
> Mental Health Financing
> Mental Health Legislation and Human Rights
> Advocacy for Mental Health
> Organization of Services for Mental Health
> Quality Improvement for Mental Health
> Planning and Budgeting to Deliver Services for Mental Health

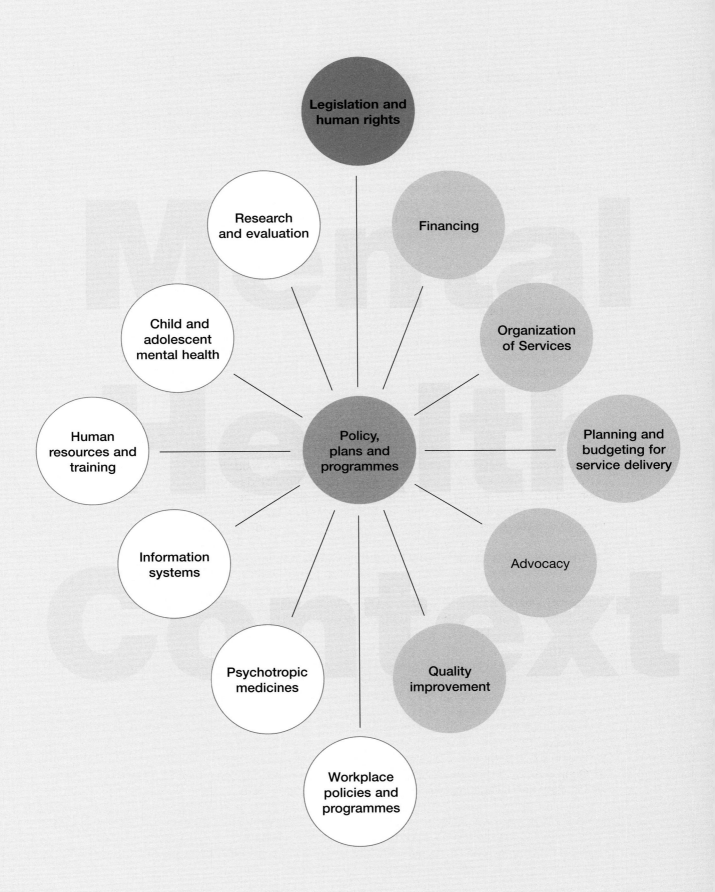

still to be developed

The following modules are not yet available but will be included in the final guidance package:

> Improving Access and Use of Psychotropic Medicines
> Mental Health Information Systems
> Human Resources and Training for Mental Health
> Child and Adolescent Mental Health
> Research and Evaluation of Mental Health Policy and Services
> Workplace Mental Health Policies and Programmes

Who is the guidance package for?

The modules will be of interest to:

- policy-makers and health planners;
- government departments at federal, state/regional and local levels;
- mental health professionals;
- groups representing people with mental disorders;
- representatives or associations of families and carers of people with mental disorders;
- advocacy organizations representing the interests of people with mental disorders and their relatives and families;
- nongovernmental organizations involved or interested in the provision of mental health services.

How to use the modules

- They can be used **individually or as a package**. They are cross-referenced with each other for ease of use. Countries may wish to go through each of the modules systematically or may use a specific module when the emphasis is on a particular area of mental health. For example, countries wishing to address mental health legislation may find the module entitled Mental Health Legislation and Human Rights useful for this purpose.

- They can be used as a **training package** for mental health policy-makers, planners and others involved in organizing, delivering and funding mental health services. They can be used as educational materials in university or college courses. Professional organizations may choose to use the package as an aid to training for persons working in mental health.

- They can be used as a framework for **technical consultancy** by a wide range of international and national organizations that provide support to countries wishing to reform their mental health policy and/or services.

- They can be used as **advocacy tools** by consumer, family and advocacy organizations. The modules contain useful information for public education and for increasing awareness among politicians, opinion-makers, other health professionals and the general public about mental disorders and mental health services.

Format of the modules

Each module clearly outlines its aims and the target audience for which it is intended. The modules are presented in a step-by-step format so as to assist countries in using and implementing the guidance provided. The guidance is not intended to be prescriptive or to be interpreted in a rigid way: countries are encouraged to adapt the material in accordance with their own needs and circumstances. Practical examples are given throughout.

There is extensive cross-referencing between the modules. Readers of one module may need to consult another (as indicated in the text) should they wish further guidance.

All the modules should be read in the light of WHO's policy of providing most mental health care through general health services and community settings. Mental health is necessarily an intersectoral issue involving the education, employment, housing, social services and criminal justice sectors. It is important to engage in serious consultation with consumer and family organizations in the development of policy and the delivery of services.

Dr Michelle Funk   Dr Benedetto Saraceno

MENTAL HEALTH LEGISLATION & HUMAN RIGHTS

Context of mental health legislation

Mental health legislation is necessary for protecting the rights of people with mental disorders, who are a vulnerable section of society. They face stigma, discrimination and marginalization in all societies, and this increases the likelihood that their human rights will be violated. Mental disorders can sometimes affect people's decision-making capacities and they may not always seek or accept treatment for their problems. Rarely, people with mental disorders may pose a risk to themselves and others because of impaired decision-making abilities. The risk of violence or harm associated with mental disorders is relatively small. Common misconceptions on this matter should not be allowed to influence mental health legislation.

Mental health legislation can provide a legal framework for addressing critical issues such as the community integration of persons with mental disorders, the provision of care of high quality, the improvement of access to care, the protection of civil rights and the protection and promotion of rights in other critical areas such as housing, education and employment. Legislation can also play an important role in promoting mental health and preventing mental disorders. Mental health legislation is thus more than care and treatment legislation that is narrowly limited to the provision of treatment in institution-based health services.

There is no national mental health legislation in 25% of countries with nearly 31% of the world's population, although countries with a federal system of governance may have state mental health laws. Of the countries in which there is mental health legislation, half have national laws that were passed after 1990. Some 15% have legislation that was enacted before 1960, i.e. before most of the currently used treatment modalities became available (World Health Organization, 2001). The existence of mental health legislation does not necessarily guarantee the protection of the human rights of people with mental disorders. In some countries, indeed, mental health legislation contains provisions that lead to the violation of human rights.

Legislation for protecting the rights of people with mental disorders may be either consolidated or dispersed. Most countries have consolidated mental health legislation, in which all the relevant issues are incorporated in a single legislative document. This has the advantage of ease of adoption and enactment. Moreover, the process of drafting, adopting and implementing such legislation provides a good opportunity for raising public awareness and educating policy-makers and society in general. The alternative is to insert provisions related to mental disorders into other legislation. For example, legislative provisions for protecting the employment rights of persons with mental disorders could be inserted in relevant employment legislation. This approach can increase the possibility of implementing provisions for the benefit of persons with mental disorders because the provisions are part of legislation that benefits a much wider range of people. However, such dispersed legislation is difficult to enact as it requires amendments and changes to multiple legislative documents. Moreover, the potential exists for important issues to be omitted.

A combined approach is most likely to address the complexity of the needs of people with mental disorders, i.e. specific mental health legislation can be complemented by more general legislation in which mental health issues are addressed.

Mental health legislation should be viewed as a process rather than as an event that occurs just once in many decades. This allows it to be amended in response to advances in the treatment of mental disorders and to developments in service delivery systems. However, frequent amendments to legislation are not feasible because of the time and financial resources required and the need to consult all stakeholders. A possible solution is to lay down regulations that are separate from legislation but can be enforced through it. Legislation can include provision for the establishment of regulations and can outline the procedure for modifying them. The most important advantage of regulations is that they do not require lawmakers to be repeatedly voting for amendments. In some countries, executive decrees and service orders are used as an alternative to regulations.

Mental health legislation is essential for complementing and reinforcing mental health policy and providing a legal framework for meeting its goals. Such legislation can protect human rights, enhance the quality of mental health services and promote the integration of persons with mental disorders into communities. These goals are an integral part of national mental health policies.

Activities preceding the formulation of legislation

Countries that have decided to draft and enact new mental health legislation have to carry out certain preliminary activities that can usefully inform this process. Firstly, it is important to identify the principal mental health problems and barriers to the implementation of mental health policies and plans. The next task is to critically review existing legislation in order to identify gaps and difficulties that can be addressed by new legislation.

An important part of these preliminary activities involves studying international human rights and the conventions and standards associated with them. Countries that are signatories to such conventions are obliged to respect, protect and fulfil the rights enshrined in them. International human rights standards such as the Principles for the Protection of Persons with Mental Illness and for the Improvement of Mental Health Care (MI Principles), the Standard Rules for Equalization of Opportunities for Persons with Disabilities (Standard Rules), the Declaration of Caracas, the Declaration of Madrid and other standards, e.g. WHO's Mental health care law: ten basic principles, can usefully inform the content of mental health legislation. These human rights standards are not legally binding on countries, but they reflect international agreement on good practice in the field of mental health.

The preliminary activities should also include a critical review of existing mental health legislation in other countries, especially ones with similar social and cultural backgrounds. This review gives a good idea of the provisions generally included in legislation in different countries. It enables the identification of provisions that limit or violate the human rights of persons with mental disorders and which, therefore, should be avoided in proposed legislation. Such a review can also lead to the identification of deficiencies that hinder the implementation of mental health legislation.

The final step in the preliminary activities is to engage all stakeholders in consultation and negotiation about possible components of mental health legislation. Consultation and negotiation for change are important not only in the drafting of legislation but also in its implementation once it has been adopted.

Content of mental health legislation

The key components of mental health legislation are discussed below. They are neither exclusive nor exhaustive but represent the most important issues that should be adequately addressed in legislation.

Substantive provisions in mental health legislation

The principle of the least restrictive alternative requires that persons are always offered treatment in settings that have the least possible effect on their personal freedom and their status and privileges in the community, including their ability to continue to work, move about and conduct their affairs. In practice, this means promoting community-based treatments and using institutional treatment settings only in rare circumstances. If institutional treatment is necessary, the legislation should encourage voluntary admission and treatment and allow involuntary admission and treatment only in exceptional circumstances. The development of community-based treatment facilities is a prerequisite for putting this principle into practice.

The legislation should guarantee to persons with mental disorders that confidentiality exists in respect of all information obtained in a clinical context. The laws should explicitly prevent disclosure, examination or transmission of patients' mental health records without their consent.

The principle of free and informed consent to treatment should be enshrined in the legislation. Treatment without consent (involuntary treatment) should be permitted only under exceptional circumstances (which must be outlined). The legislation should incorporate adequate procedural mechanisms that protect the rights of persons with mental disorders who are being treated involuntarily, and should permit clinical and research trials only if patients have given free and informed consent. This applies equally to patients admitted involuntarily to mental health facilities and to voluntary patients.

Involuntary admission to hospital should be the exception and should happen only in very specific circumstances. The legislation should outline these exceptional circumstances and lay down the procedures to be followed for involuntary admission. The legislation should give patients who are admitted involuntarily the right of appeal against their admission to a review body.

Voluntary treatment is associated with the issue of informed consent. The legislation should ensure that all treatments are provided on the basis of free and informed consent except in rare circumstances. Consent cannot be lawful if accompanied by a threat or implied threat of compulsion, or if alternatives to proposed treatment are not offered for consideration.

The legislation should only permit voluntary treatment, i.e. after informed consent has been obtained, of patients admitted voluntarily to mental health facilities. Involuntary patients should also be treated on a voluntary basis except in certain rare situations, e.g. if they lack the capacity to give consent and if treatment is necessary in order to improve mental health and/or prevent a significant deterioration in mental health and/or prevent injury or harm to the patients or other people. The legislation should lay down procedures for protecting the human rights of people who are being treated involuntarily and should provide them with protection against harm and the misuse of the powers indicated above. These procedures include obtaining an independent second opinion, obtaining permission from an independent authority based on professional recommendations, giving patients access to the right to appeal against involuntary treatment, and using a periodic review mechanism.

Involuntary treatment in community settings (community supervision) can be a useful alternative to admission to institutions and can conform to the principle of the least restrictive alternative. An evaluation of the effectiveness of community supervision is not possible because there is still insufficient evidence and knowledge in this field. However, in countries that have adopted community supervision it is important that sufficient measures exist to protect the human rights of the patients concerned, as in other treatment settings.

The legislation should make provisions for the automatic reviewing of all instances of involuntary admission and involuntary treatment. This should involve an independent review body with legal or quasi-legal status enabling it to act as a regulatory authority. The legislation should specify the composition, powers and duties of such a body.

The legislation should make provision for the appointment of guardians of persons who are not competent to make decisions and manage their own affairs. The procedures for making competence decisions, including the appropriate authority for such decisions and the duties of guardians and protective mechanisms to prevent the abuse of powers by guardians, should be specified in legislation.

Substantive provisions for other legislation impacting on mental health

The components of legislation concerning sectors outside the health sector are also important for the prevention of mental disorders and the promotion of mental health. Housing is of tremendous importance in relation to the integration of persons with mental disorders into communities. Housing legislation should protect the rights of persons with mental disorders, for example by preventing geographical segregation, giving them priority in state housing schemes and mandating local authorities to establish a range of housing facilities.

Children, youth and adults have the right to suitable educational opportunities and facilities. Countries should ensure that the education of people with mental disorders is an integral part of their educational systems. Specific mental health programmes in schools have a role to play in the early identification of emotional and behavioural problems in children and can thus help to prevent disabilities attributable to mental disorders. School-based programmes also help to increase awareness about emotional and behavioural disorders and to develop skills for coping with adversity and stress.

Employment is a key area for the promotion of community integration. The legislation should protect persons with mental disorders from discrimination, exploitation and unfair dismissal from work on grounds of mental disorder. There is also a need for legislation to promote the establishment and funding of vocational rehabilitation programmes, including the provision of preferential financing and affirmative action programmes.

Disability pensions and benefits are another area where legislation can help to protect and promote the rights of persons with mental disorders and further the cause of community integration. Civil legislation should enable persons with mental disorders to exercise all their civil, political, economic, social and cultural rights, including the rights to vote, marry, have children, own property and have freedom of movement and choice of residence. Other areas of legislative action include the improvement of access to psychotropic medication and the provision of mental health services in primary health care.

The legislation can include specific provisions for protecting the rights of vulnerable groups such as women, children, the elderly and indigenous ethnic populations. There can be measures to promote mother-and-child bonding by the provision of maternal leave, to facilitate the early detection and prevention of child abuse, to restrict access to alcohol and drugs, and to establish mental health programmes in schools.

Process issues in mental health legislation

The task of drafting legislation should be delegated to a special committee whose composition should reflect competing ideologies. The members of the committee should bring an adequate diversity of expertise to the task. The participation of users and carers is crucially important but frequently neglected. The committee should include representatives of government ministries, legislators, mental health professionals, representatives of users, carers and advocacy organizations, and experts with experience of working with women, children, the elderly and other vulnerable groups.

The draft of proposed legislation should be presented for consultation to all the key stakeholders in the mental health field. Consultation has a key role in identifying weaknesses in proposed legislation, potential conflicts with existing legislation, key issues inadvertently left out of the draft legislation and possible practical difficulties in implementation. Consultation also provides an opportunity for raising public awareness about mental health issues. Most importantly, systematic consultation can have a positive impact on the implementation of legislation.

The process of adopting legislation is likely to be the most time-consuming step. Other priorities, especially in developing countries, may mean that mental health legislation is ignored or delayed in legislatures. The mobilizing of public opinion and the active lobbying of lawmakers are possible ways of promoting and hastening the process of adopting mental health legislation.

Difficulties in implementation can be anticipated as from the stage when legislation is being drafted, and corrective measures can then be taken. In many countries, poor attention to implementation has meant that practice differs from what is laid down in law. Implementation difficulties may arise because of a lack of finances, a shortage of human resources, a lack of awareness about mental health legislation among professionals, carers, families and the general public, a lack of coordinated action and, occasionally, procedural difficulties.

Clearly, funds are required for the implementation of new mental health legislation. For example, they are needed for the functioning of the review body, for training mental health professionals in the use of legislation and for changes to mental health services as required by legislation. Adequate budgetary provision should be made for these activities. Since mental health budgets are part of general health budgets in many countries it is important to ensure that the budgets meant for mental health are used only for this purpose and not diverted to other health issues.

A coordinating agency can help with the implementation of various sections of mental health legislation in accordance with a schedule. This role can be performed by the ministry of health with assistance from a review body and advocacy organizations. Some of the functions of the coordinating agency include developing rules and procedures for implementation, preparing standardized documentation instruments, and developing training and certification procedures for mental health professionals.

Implementation is helped by wide dissemination of the provisions of new mental health legislation among mental health professionals and users, carers and their families and advocacy organizations. A sustained programme of public education and increasing public awareness can also play an important role in implementation.

This module aims to:

- provide an overview of the context of mental health legislation and outline the key areas of content in such legislation;
- underline the steps in formulating and implementing mental health legislation;
- serve as an advocacy tool to promote the adoption and implementation of mental health legislation.

This module will be of interest to:

- policy-makers, legislators, general health planners and mental health planners;
- user groups;
- representatives or associations of families and carers of persons with mental disorders;
- advocacy organizations representing the interests of persons with mental disorders and their relatives and families;
- human rights groups working with and on behalf of persons with mental disorders;
- officials in ministries of health, social welfare and justice.

1. Introduction

1.1 Necessity of mental health legislation

Mental health legislation is essential because of the unique vulnerabilities of people with mental disorders. These vulnerabilities exist for two reasons.

Firstly, mental disorders can affect the way people think and behave, their capacity to protect their own interests and, on rare occasions, their decision-making abilities. Secondly, persons with mental disorders face stigma, discrimination and marginalization in most societies. Stigmatization increases the probability that they will not be offered the treatment they need or that they will be offered services that are of inferior quality and not sensitive to their needs. Marginalization and discrimination also increase the risk of violation of their civil, political, economic, social and cultural rights by mental health service providers and others.

People with mental disorders may, on rare occasions, pose a risk to themselves or others because of behavioural disturbances and impairments in their decision-making capacities. This has consequences for people who come into contact with them, including family members, neighbours, work colleagues and society at large. The risk of violence or harm associated with mental disorders is relatively small. Common misconceptions about the dangerousness of these disorders should not influence the thrust of mental health legislation.

People with mental disorders experience some of the harshest living conditions in many societies. They face economic marginalization, at least in part because of discrimination and the absence of legal protections against improper and abusive treatment. They are often denied opportunities to be educated, to work or to enjoy the benefits of public services or other facilities. There are many instances of laws that do not actively discriminate against people with mental disorders but place improper or unnecessary barriers or burdens on them. In some countries, people with mental disorders are subject to discrimination, i.e. the arbitrary denial of rights that are afforded to all other citizens.

Mental health legislation is thus concerned with more than care and treatment, i.e. it is not limited to the provision of institution-based health services. It provides a legal framework for addressing critical mental health issues such as access to care, the provision of care of high quality, rehabilitation and aftercare, the full integration of people with mental disorders into communities, the prevention of mental disorders and the promotion of mental health in different sectors of society.

The existence of national mental health legislation does not necessarily guarantee respect for and protection of the human rights of people with mental disorders. Indeed, in some countries the provisions of mental health legislation result in the violation of the human rights of such people. There is no national mental health legislation in 25% of countries with nearly 31% of the world's population, although countries with a federal system of governance may have state mental health laws. There are wide variations in this matter between different regions of the world. Thus 91.7% of countries in the European Region have national mental health legislation, whereas in the Eastern Mediterranean Region only 57% have such legislation. In 50% of countries, laws in this field were passed after 1990, while in 15% there is mental health legislation dating from before the 1960s, when most of today's treatment methods were unavailable (World Health Organization, 2001).

Persons with mental disorders are a vulnerable section of the population.

Persons with mental disorder face stigma in most societies.

Persons with mental disorders experience economic marginalization and discrimination.

Mental health legislation should be comprehensive.

There is no mental health legislation in 25% of countries.

1.2 Approaches to mental health legislation

There are two ways of approaching mental health legislation. In some countries there is no separate mental health legislation and provisions relating to people with mental disorders are inserted into relevant legislation in other areas. This is referred to as dispersed legislation. Most countries, however, have consolidated mental health legislation, in which all issues of relevance to people with mental disorders are incorporated into a single instrument.

Both approaches have advantages and disadvantages. Consolidated legislation is easy to enact and adopt without a need for multiple amendments of existing laws. The process of drafting, adopting and implementing consolidated legislation also provides good opportunities for raising public awareness about mental disorders and educating policy-makers and the general public about human rights issues, stigma and discrimination. However, it has been argued that consolidated legislation emphasizes the segregation of mental health issues and persons with mental disorders. It has the potential to reinforce stigma and prejudice against persons with such disorders.

The strategy of inserting provisions relating to mental disorders into relevant legislation purports to reduce stigma and emphasizes the integration of people with mental disorders into communities. Dispersed legislative provisions also increase the possibility that laws enacted for the benefit of people with mental disorders are put into practice because they are part of legislation that benefits a much wider range of people. The experience of many countries shows that practice sometimes differs from what is laid down in law about matters of mental health. The main disadvantage of dispersed legislation is the difficulty in ensuring coverage of all legislative matters of relevance to persons with mental disorders. Moreover, more legislative time is necessary because of the need for multiple amendments to existing laws.

There is little evidence to show that one approach is better than the other. A combined approach is most likely to address the complex needs of persons with mental disorders. Mental health issues should be included in other legislation, and, preferably complemented by specific mental health legislation.

Mental health legislation should not be viewed as an event but as an ongoing process that evolves with time. This means that legislation should be reviewed, revised and amended in the light of advances in the treatment of mental disorders and improvements in service development and delivery. It is difficult to specify the frequency with mental health legislation should be amended. However, a period of five to ten years seems appropriate, taking into account the experience of countries that have made amendments in this field, e.g. the United Kingdom. In reality, it is difficult to make frequent amendments to legislation because of the length of the process, the costs and the need to consult all stakeholders.

One solution is to make provision for the introduction of regulations for particular actions that are likely to need constant modification. Regulations are not written into the legislation, which simply outlines the process for introducing and reviewing them. In South Africa, for example, mental health legislation makes extensive use of regulations. Rules for the accreditation of mental health professionals are not written into the legislation but are part of the regulations. The legislation specifies who is responsible for framing regulations and indicates the broad principles on which regulations are based. The advantage of using regulations in this way is that frequent modification of the accreditation rules is possible without a lengthy process of amending primary legislation. Regulations thus lend an element of flexibility to mental health legislation. Executive decrees and service orders are used as alternatives to regulations in some countries.

Most countries have consolidated legislation.

Consolidated legislation is easy to enact and adopt.

Dispersed legislation can help to reduce stigma and emphasize community integration.

A combined approach of dispersed and consolidated legislation is preferable.

Mental health legislation should be viewed as a process rather than as an event.

Regulations can be used as part of legislation.

1.3 Interface between mental health policy and legislation

Mental health legislation is essential to complement and reinforce mental health policy and is not a substitute for it. It provides a legal framework ensuring the consideration of critical issues such as access to mental health care, the provision of care that is humane and of high quality, rehabilitation and aftercare, the full integration of persons with mental disorders into the community and the promotion of mental health in different sectors of society.

Legislation provides a legal framework for achieving the goals of mental health policy.

Among the key aspects of the interface between policy and legislation are the following.

1.3.1 **Human rights.** Human rights should be an integral dimension of the design, implementation, monitoring and evaluation of mental health policies and programmes. They include, but are not limited to, the rights to: equality and non-discrimination; dignity and respect; privacy and individual autonomy; and information and participation. Mental health legislation is a tool for codifying and consolidating these fundamental values and principles of mental health policy.

Legislation codifies the values and principles of human rights which are embedded in mental health policy.

1.3.2 **Community integration.** This is important in nearly all countries that have recently developed or revised their mental health policies. Legislation can ensure that involuntary admission is restricted to rare situations in which individuals pose a threat to themselves and/or others and community based alternatives are considered unfeasible. It can therefore create incentives for the development of a range of community-based facilities and services. The restriction of involuntary admission to a limited period of time, usually months rather than years, creates further incentives for community-based care and rehabilitation. Legislation allows people with mental disorders and their families and carers to play an important role in interactions with mental health services, including admission to mental health facilities. For example, people can appeal on behalf of members of their families and they have the right to be consulted on the planning of treatment. The legislation can thus help to maintain social networks and links that are crucial for community integration. These links have been shown to affect outcomes: in a study of 226 patients in a long-term care unit in Nigeria the discontinuation of visits from members of extended families contributed to long or indefinite stays by patients (Jegede et al., 1985).

Legislation can help to promote the integration into communities of persons with mental disorders.

1.3.3 **Links with other sectors.** Legislation can prevent discrimination against persons with mental disorders in the area of employment. Examples include protection from dismissal on account of mental disorders and affirmative action programmes to improve access to paid employment. With regard to housing, legislation can improve access by preventing the geographical segregation of persons with mental disorders and mandating local authorities to provide subsidized housing to people disabled by such disorders. Legislation on disability pensions can also promote equity and fairness.

Legislation can help to achieve the aims of mental health policy in areas outside the mental health sector.

1.3.4 **Enhancing the quality of care.** Legislative provisions on general living conditions and protection against inhuman and degrading treatment can lead to significant improvements in the built environment of mental health facilities. Legislation can set minimum standards in respect of treatment and living conditions for the accreditation of mental health facilities. It can lay down minimum qualifications and skills for the accreditation of mental health professionals, thus ensuring that a basic minimum level of expertise is provided throughout the country in question. It can also set minimum staffing standards for the accreditation of mental health facilities and can therefore act as a major incentive for investment in the development of human resources.

Legislation can help to enhance the quality of care.

Key points: Introduction

- People with mental disorders constitute a vulnerable section of society.

- Mental health legislation is necessary for protecting the rights of people with mental disorders.

- Mental health legislation is concerned with more than care and treatment. It provides a legal framework to address critical mental health issues such as access to care, rehabilitation and aftercare, full integration of people with mental disorders into the community, and the promotion of mental health in different sectors of society.

- There is no national mental health legislation is in 25% of countries with nearly 31% of the world's population.

- Legislative issues pertaining to mental health can be consolidated into a single instrument or dispersed in different documents. A combination of both approaches is likely to be the most effective solution.

- Mental health legislation is an integral part of mental health policy and provides a legislative framework for achieving the goals of such policy.

2. Preliminary activities to be undertaken by countries wishing to formulate mental health legislation

Before the process of drafting and adopting legislation begins, certain activities that can usefully inform decisions on its content have to be undertaken. These activities include the following:

(1) Identifying the principal mental disorders and barriers to the implementation of policy and programmes in the country concerned;

(2) Identifying (or mapping) existing mental health laws or general laws that address mental health issues and looking for legal aspects that are lacking or in need of reformulation;

(3) Studying international conventions and standards related to human rights and mental health and identifying obligations and internationally accepted norms under international human rights instruments that have been ratified by the country;

(4) Studying components of mental health legislation in other countries, especially countries with similar social and cultural backgrounds;

(5) Consulting and negotiating for change.

In most countries the professionals in charge of mental health in the ministries of health will take responsibility for these preliminary activities.

Professionals in ministries of health should take responsibility for preliminary activities.

2.1 Identifying the country's principal mental disorders and barriers to implementation of policy and programmes

The first step is to obtain reliable information about mental disorders in the whole country and about variations between different regions and population groups. This information is usually gathered during the development of national mental health policies and plans. Through this process it will therefore be available to those working on mental health legislation. (See Mental Health Policy, Plans and Programmes and Planning and Budgeting to Deliver Services for Mental Health.)

It is also important to form a clear understanding of the barriers to implementation of mental health policies and programmes. The legislation can be used to overcome or break down some of these barriers, especially those relating to access and equity. Box 1 lists some of the barriers that can be tackled by legislative efforts and gives an indication of priority areas for legislation.

Box 1. Principal barriers to the development of mental health policies and programmes which legislation can help to overcome

- There may be a lack of mental health services in some areas or in the country as a whole.

- The cost of mental health care may be unaffordable to many people, and health insurance may include only partial coverage for psychiatric treatments or none at all.

- The quality of care and the living conditions in mental hospitals may be poor, leading to human rights violations.

- Regulations and checks concerning involuntary admission and treatment are usually lacking, and this is often associated with loss of liberty.

- Stigma and discrimination associated with mental disorders impact negatively on access to care and on the social integration of people suffering from such disorders.

- Persons with mental disorders may be denied basic rights in respect of civil matters, social participation, cultural expression, participation in elections, freedom of opinion, housing, employment, education and other areas.

- Some social conditions or cultural practices may damage the mental health of certain population groups.

- There may be a lack of resources for mental health programmes in schools and workplaces.

2.2 Mapping of legislation related to mental health

The next task is to identify existing mental health legislation and components of general laws as they relate to people with mental disorders. A systematic and critical review of such legislation will identify lacunae and difficulties that should be addressed by new legislation. Such a review may also reveal that existing legislative documents do not have adequate provisions for ensuring care of satisfactory quality and protecting the rights of people with mental disorders. Occasionally, it will be found that countries have adequate provisions in existing legislation and that there is a problem of implementation. In these cases, there may be little need to alter, modify or amend legislation or introduce new legislation. (See Section 6.)

The next task is to review existing legislation in order to identify areas that should be addressed by new legislation.

2.3 Studying international conventions and standards

Countries that have signed international human rights conventions are obliged to respect, protect and fulfil the rights enshrined in them. Among the most important of these conventions are the International Bill of Rights, which includes the United Nations Declaration of Human Rights, the International Covenant on Civil and Political Rights and the International Covenant on Economic, Social and Cultural Rights. It is therefore important that these instruments are reviewed thoroughly when mental health legislation is being planned. There are also agreed international standards of good practice which are not legally binding. These include the Principles for the Protection of Persons with Mental Illness and for the Improvement of Mental Health Care (MI Principles), the Standard Rules for Equalization of Opportunities for Persons with Disabilities, the Declaration of Caracas, the Declaration of Madrid and other standards such as WHO's *Mental health care law: ten basic principles*.

Several international conventions and standards should inform countries' legislation.

Certain international covenants, although not specifically designed for the protection of persons with mental disorders, provide legally enforceable protection of human rights in signatory countries. For example, Article 7 of the International Covenant on Civil and Political Rights provides all individuals, including those with mental disorders, protection from torture and cruel, inhuman or degrading treatment or punishment as well as the right not to be subjected to medical or scientific experimentation without informed consent. Article 12 of the International Covenant on Economic, Social and Cultural Rights recognizes the right of everyone, including people with mental disorders, to the enjoyment of the highest attainable standard of physical and mental health.

Certain international covenants provide legally enforceable protection of human rights.

The European Convention for Protection of Human Rights and Fundamental Freedoms, backed by the European Court of Human Rights, provides more binding protection for the human rights of persons with mental disorders residing in the countries that have ratified it. Mental health legislation in European countries has to provide for safeguards against the involuntary admission of persons with mental disorders on the basis of the three following principles laid down by the European Court of Human Rights: a) mental disorder has to be established by objective medical expertise; b) mental disorder has to be of a nature and degree warranting compulsory confinement; c) the persistence of mental disorder has to be proved in order to justify continued confinement (Wachenfield, 1992).

There are several regional covenants on human rights, such as those in Europe, the Americas and Africa.

Mental health legislation in European countries is also influenced by Recommendation 1235 on Psychiatry and Human Rights (1994) adopted by the Parliamentary Assembly of the Council of Europe, which lays down criteria for the involuntary admission of persons with mental disorders, the procedure for making decisions on involuntary admission, standards for care and treatment given to persons with mental disorders, and prohibitions aimed at preventing abuses in psychiatric care and practice.

In the Region of the Americas, a combination of instruments affords protection of human rights to all persons, including those with mental disorders. These instruments include the American Declaration of the Rights and Duties of Man, the American Convention on Human Rights, the Additional Protocol to the American Convention on Human Rights in the area of economic, social and cultural rights, and the Inter-American Convention on the Elimination of all Forms of Discrimination against Persons with Disabilities.

The American Declaration of the Rights and Duties of Man is a non-binding document that covers the protection of civil, political, economic, social and cultural rights. The American Convention on Human Rights explicitly states that every person has the right to physical, mental and moral integrity, that no one shall be subject to cruel, inhuman or degrading punishment and treatment and that all persons deprived of their liberty shall be treated with the inherent dignity of the human person.

The Additional Protocol to the American Convention on Human Rights provides further protection for people with mental disorders, stating that, in order to achieve the full exercise of the right to education, programmes of special education should be established so as to provide special instruction and training for persons with physical disabilities or mental deficiencies. It also states that all persons affected by a diminution of their physical or mental capacities are entitled to receive special attention to help them to achieve the greatest possible development of their personality, and that everyone has the right to social security to protect them from the consequences of old age and disability which prevent them, physically or mentally, from securing the means for a dignified and decent existence.

The Inter-American Convention on the Elimination of all Forms of Discrimination against Persons with Disabilities has not yet come into force. Its objectives are to prevent and eliminate all forms of discrimination against persons with mental or physical disabilities and to promote their full integration into society. It is the first international convention specifically addressing the rights of persons with mental disorders.

Another example of a regional mechanism for the protection of human rights is the African (Banjul) Charter on Human and People's Rights, a legally binding document supervised by the African Commission on Human and People's Rights. Article 16 guarantees the right to enjoy the best attainable state of physical and mental health, Article 4 covers the right to life and the integrity of the person, and Article 5 concerns the right to respect for the dignity inherent in human beings and the prohibition of all forms of exploitation and degradation, particularly slavery, slave trade, torture and cruel, inhuman or degrading punishment and treatment.

An increasing awareness of disability caused by and related to mental disorders has led to a move away from an illness paradigm and towards a disability paradigm for understanding the social consequences of mental disorders. Understanding these disorders in terms of disability leads to further legislative opportunities to protect the rights of the affected persons. For example, United Nations Resolution 48/96 on Standard Rules for the Equalization of Opportunities for Persons with Disabilities (1993) aims to ensure equal opportunities and protect the rights of disabled persons. Disability-related legislation arising from the implementation of these Standard Rules can provide a second tier of protection against violation of the human rights of persons with mental disorders.

There is an increased move towards a disability paradigm for understanding the consequences of mental disorders.

International agencies and organizations have attempted to guide national mental health legislation by developing standards and guidelines for protecting the rights of persons with mental disorders. Although these guidelines are not directly enforceable, they represent international opinion on the essential components of mental health legislation.

Standards and guidelines have also been developed in order to protect the rights of people with mental disorders.

In 1991 the United Nations General Assembly adopted Resolution 46/119, comprising principles for protecting the human rights of persons with mental disorders. The Principles for the Protection of Persons with Mental Illness and for the Improvement of Mental Health Care bring together a set of basic rights that the international community regards as inviolable in community and treatment settings. The 25 principles cover the following areas:

- definition of mental illness;
- protection of confidentiality;
- standards of care and treatment, including involuntary admission and consent to treatment;
- rights of persons with mental disorders in mental health facilities;
- protection of minors;
- provision of resources for mental health facilities;
- role of community and culture;
- review mechanisms providing for the protection of the rights of offenders with mental disorders;
- procedural safeguards protecting the rights of persons with mental disorders.

In order to facilitate the understanding and implementation of the United Nations Principles, WHO published guidelines to the human rights of persons with mental disorders (World Health Organization, 1996a). The guidelines include a checklist to facilitate the rapid assessment of human rights conditions at the local and regional levels. A further document that aids the implementation of the United Nations Principles is entitled *Mental health care law: ten basic principles* (World Health Organization, 1996b). It is based on a comparative analysis of national mental health laws and describes ten basic principles for mental health legislation irrespective of the cultural or legal context. There are annotations on the implementation of the principles. (See Box 2.)

The Declaration of Caracas, adopted by the Regional Conference on Restructuring Psychiatric Care in Latin America in 1990, is an example of regional collaboration for the protection of the rights of persons with mental disorders. This Declaration aims to promote community-based integrated mental health services by restructuring psychiatric care involving services provided in mental hospitals. The Declaration states that resources, care and treatment for persons with mental disorders should safeguard their dignity and human and civil rights, provide rational and appropriate treatment and strive to maintain such persons in their communities. It further states that mental health legislation should safeguard the human rights of persons with mental disorders and that services should be organized so that these rights can be enforced.

International associations of mental health professionals have also endeavoured to ensure the human rights of persons with mental disorders by issuing guidelines for standards of professional behaviour and practice. Such guidelines are contained, for example, in the Declaration of Madrid, adopted in 1996 by the General Assembly of the World Psychiatric Association. Among other standards the Declaration insists on treatment based on partnership with persons who have mental disorders and on the enforcement of involuntary treatment only under exceptional circumstances.

The United Nations has adopted principles for the protection of people with mental illness and the improvement of mental health care.

Mental health care law: ten basic principles.

Declaration of Caracas.

Declaration of Madrid.

Box 2. Mental health care law: ten basic principles
(World Health Organization, 1996b)

- Promotion of mental health and prevention of mental disorders
- Access to basic mental health care
- Mental health assessment in accordance with internationally accepted principles
- Provision of the least restrictive type of mental health care
- Self-determination
- Right to be assisted in the exercise of self-determination
- Availability of review procedures
- Automatic periodic review mechanism
- Qualified decision-makers
- Respect for the rule of law

2.4 Reviewing mental health legislation in other countries

Reviewing other countries' legislation related to mental health gives a good idea of the components that are generally included. A review can identify useful components that are protective of human rights as well as provisions that limit or violate human rights and should therefore be avoided in proposed legislation.

The review should also critically examine the extent to which legislation can improve the situation for people with mental disorders in the countries concerned. Reasons for failure should be identified. They might include: (1) badly drafted legislation that does not include provisions for protecting the rights of people with mental disorders, adequately addressing their needs, or promoting access to satisfactory care; (2) difficulties of implementation which arise because stakeholders refuse to cooperate; (3) legislative provisions that do not take account of practical realities. (See Section 3.1.4 and example from South Africa in Section 8).

Some of the main components of mental health legislation in countries in different regions of the world are listed in Box 3, which can be used as a general framework enabling the identification of specific components in particular countries. The list is not meant to be an exhaustive compilation of all the necessary components of mental health legislation.

Reviewing other countries' legislation gives a good idea of the components that are generally included.

Box 3. Substantive provisions of legislation for mental health

Mental health legislation	Other legislation influencing mental health
Protecting rights	Protecting rights, promotion and prevention

- Access to basic mental health care - Least restrictive care - Informed consent to treatment - Voluntary and involuntary admission and treatment - Competence issues - Periodical review mechanism - Confidentiality - Rehabilitation - Accreditation of professionals and facilities - Rights of families and carers	- Housing - Education - Employment - Social security - Criminal justice - General health care - Affirmative action - Rehabilitation, including vocational services - Detection of child abuse - Restrictions on access to alcohol and drugs - Protection of vulnerable groups - Civil legislation

2.5 Consultation and negotiating for change

The activities mentioned above can help decision-making with regard to the components to be included in new legislation and the amendments and modifications to be made in existing legislation. Consultation and negotiation with all stakeholders on these matters constitute an important next step in this process. The stakeholders include: people with mental disorders and their representative organizations; carers and families of persons with mental disorders; professionals, including psychiatrists, psychologists, psychiatric nurses and social workers; politicians; policy-makers; government ministries (health, social welfare, law, finance); advocacy organizations; service providers including non-governmental organizations; civil rights groups and religious organizations.

Consultation and negotiation are important not only in the drafting of legislation but also in ensuring that it is implemented once it has been adopted. Consultation and negotiation provide an opportunity to address misconceptions, misapprehensions and fears about mental disorders. The language of human rights provides a counterweight to the practices of exclusion and stigmatization.

Consultation and negotiation play an important role in drafting, adopting and, most importantly, implementing new mental health

Key points: Preliminary activities

- Legislation can help to overcome some of the barriers to the implementation of mental health policies and programmes, especially those related to access and equity.

- A systematic and critical review of existing legislation can identify lacunae and difficulties to be addressed by proposed legislation.

- Countries that have signed international human rights conventions are obliged to protect, respect and fulfil the rights enshrined in them. It is therefore important that these instruments are reviewed thoroughly when mental health legislation is being planned.

- International standards such as those in the MI Principles, the Standard Rules and Mental health care law: ten basic principles, although not legally binding, represent international agreement on standards of good practice.

- Reviews of other countries' legislation can highlight the provisions commonly found in mental health laws. They can also identify provisions that should be avoided in proposed legislation because they limit or violate the human rights of people with mental disorders. Furthermore, they may identify reasons for the failure of such legislation to improve the situation of persons with mental disorders in the country concerned.

- Consultation and negotiation with all stakeholders on the possible components of mental health legislation and amendments to existing legislation provide an opportunity to address misconceptions, misapprehensions and fears relating to mental disorders, and tend to favour the successful implementation of such legislation.

3. Key components of mental health legislation

This section discusses the key areas that should be included in mental health legislation. These components are neither exclusive nor exhaustive but represent some of the most important issues to address if the legislation is to be adequate. For a more comprehensive listing, see the Principles for the Protection of Persons with Mental Illness and for the Improvement of Mental Health Care (MI Principles) and *Guidelines for the promotion of human rights of persons with mental disorders* (World Health Organization, 1996a).

Legislation aimed at protecting the rights of people with mental disorders should not be restricted to issues of mental health or even of general health. Other areas of relevance which are not strictly health-related but which are of enormous importance include those of employment, education and housing legislation. These and other such issues are discussed below. (See Section 3.2.)

Legislation that is concerned with mental health should not be restricted to the health sector.

Countries intending to formulate comprehensive legislation that covers all issues of relevance to people with mental disorders may wish to include the provisions in a single instrument. Other countries may already have legislation covering certain matters in this field and may prefer to make amendments to legislative documents in order to protect the rights of persons with mental disorders. Legislation in areas that affect mental health but that are not necessarily included in mental health legislation is described at the end of this section. These areas are vital to the welfare of persons with mental disorders and should therefore receive adequate legislative attention. They are also important in the promotion of mental health and the prevention of mental disorders.

3.1 Substantive provisions for mental health legislation

3.1.1 The principle of the least restrictive alternative

All people with mental disorders should be provided with treatment based in the community except in very rare circumstances, e.g. if there is a risk of self-harm or of harm to other people or if the treatment can only be provided in an institutional setting. If institutional admission or treatment is necessary, legislation should encourage this on a voluntary basis. Laws should permit involuntary admission and treatment only in exceptional circumstances. If involuntary admission does happen there should be procedures for protecting the rights of the persons concerned.

In particular, a number of criteria should be met before involuntary admission or treatment takes place. Firstly, qualified mental health professionals with legal authorization should determine that the person in question has a mental disorder. Secondly, they should be convinced that the mental disorder represents a high probability of immediate or imminent harm to this person or other persons, or, in the case of a person whose mental disorder is severe and whose judgement is impaired, that failure to admit or detain the person would probably lead to a serious deterioration in her or his condition or would prevent appropriate treatment such as could only be administered by admission to a mental health facility.

In countries where community-based treatment is minimal or unavailable, efforts and resources should be directed towards the establishment and strengthening of services in order to make alternatives to admission as widely available as possible.

Mental health care law: ten basic principles (World Health Organization, 1996b) states that any legal instruments that include provisions incompatible with community-based mental health care should be removed. In order to ensure effective implementation of the principle of the least restrictive alternative it states there should be legal instruments and infrastructures to support community-based mental health care involving settings suitable for patients with various degrees of autonomy.

People should be offered the least restrictive treatments.

3.1.2 Confidentiality

There should be legislative provisions ensuring that all information and records about a person's mental disorders are kept confidential. Laws should explicitly prevent the disclosure, examination or transmission of a patient's mental health records without her or his consent and/or the consent of a legally appointed representative or guardian. Similarly, legislation should require professionals to obtain consent before disclosing any non-written information obtained during the assessment or treatment of mental disorders.

The legislation should protect the confidentiality of all information obtained in a clinical context.

It is also important to take into account the needs of carers and families. Appropriate and adequate information should be available to them so that they can provide proper care for patients living at home. Legislation should attempt to strike a fine balance between the principle of confidentiality and the needs of carers and families for information in order that patients can be looked after appropriately.

There are, however, specific and rare exceptions to the principle of confidentiality. For example, a professional may be justified in breaking confidentiality if there is imminent danger of harm to the person in question or to other persons. Moreover, in a criminal trial the court may order professionals to reveal information and/or records of mental disorders. Mental health legislation in most countries recognizes the rights of courts to override confidentiality in criminal cases but not in civil cases (e.g. divorce, property matters). The legislation should clearly delineate the circumstances in which confidentiality can be set aside and should include adequate safeguards against the misuse and abuse of this provision.

There are certain rare exceptions to the requirement for confidentiality.

3.1.3 Informed consent

The principle of free and informed consent is the cornerstone of treatment for mental disorders and should therefore be enshrined in mental health legislation. The key issue regarding consent for treatment lies in establishing the patient's competence to give consent. The right to give consent to treatment is accompanied by the right to refuse it. If a patient is judged competent to give consent, her or his refusal to accept treatment also has to be respected.

Informed consent is the cornerstone of treatment for mental disorders.

To be valid, consent must satisfy the following criteria (MI Principles and Guidelines to MI Principles).

a) The person/patient giving consent should be judged competent and able to give consent.
b) Consent should be obtained freely, without threats or improper inducements.
c) There should be appropriate and adequate disclosure of information on the purpose, method, likely duration and expected benefits of the proposed treatment.
d) Possible pain or discomfort, risks and the likely side-effects of the proposed treatment should be adequately discussed with the patient.
e) Choices should be offered. Alternative modes of treatment, especially ones that are less intrusive should be discussed and offered to the patient.

There are several criteria for informed consent.

f) Information should be provided in a language
and form that is understandable to the patient.
g) The patient should have the right to refuse or stop treatment.
h) The consequences of refusing treatment should
be explained to the patient.

In exceptional circumstances, the legislation may allow treatment to proceed without informed consent. This may happen, for example, if a person has a severe mental disorder, is found to be lacking competence (capacity) and treatment is likely to alleviate the disorder or there is a likelihood of further deterioration of the patient's condition if treatment is not given. (See Section 3.1.5.)

In exceptional circumstances, treatment may be allowed without informed consent.

The legislation should not permit participation in clinical or experimental research without informed consent, which must be obtained from all patients, whether voluntarily or involuntarily admitted.

Many jurisdictions use age (usually 18 years) as the sole criterion for determining the right of minors to give consent or refuse consent. However, a significant number of minors, especially teenagers, are sufficiently mature and understanding to be able to give or withhold consent. There should be provisions in the legislation to encourage the relevant professionals to take minors' opinions into consideration in matters of consent, depending on their age and maturity.

The consent of minors is an important issue for legislation.

3.1.4 Voluntary and involuntary admission

The laws should encourage voluntary admission and, in exceptional circumstances, should permit involuntary admission. Where there is a potential for involuntary admission, this should only be used in very specific circumstances and in accordance with the law. Public misconceptions about the dangerousness of people with mental disorders lead to undue emphasis on protecting society from the risk of violence and harm. The law should be seen as striking a balance between the right of the individual to self-determination and personal responsibility on one hand and the ability of the state to promote the safety and welfare of the individual and the wider community on the other.

Legislation should promote voluntary admission to mental health facilities.

In this connection the key issue involves outlining circumstances in which involuntary admission is considered appropriate and laying down the procedure for invoking powers for involuntary admission. Involuntary admission is permitted only if **both** the following criteria are met:

Involuntary admission should only be used in exceptional circumstances.

- there is evidence of mental disorder of specified severity as defined
by internationally accepted standards;
- there is a likelihood of self-harm or harm to others and/or of a deterioration
in the patient's condition if treatment is not given.

The circumstances in the country in question should also be considered when provisions for involuntary admission are being framed. A good example of this is legislative provision for certification from at least two psychiatrists before involuntary admission to hospital takes place. The purpose of such provision is to give adequate protection against compulsory admission. However, low-income countries with few psychiatrists find it extremely difficult to implement this kind of provision. In many cases, such provision remains ignored and professionals and family members continue with existing practices for involuntary admission. In these circumstances, a better option would be to request certification by two doctors or two mental health professionals, of whom at least one should be a psychiatrist. Where there is a shortage of psychiatrists it may be necessary for other professionals to undertake the assessment and make the decisions. These professionals could be social workers, psychologists or nurses who have received the required training. This increases the pool of mental health professionals available to provide certification and helps to meet the need for adequate protection of persons with mental disorders. (See example from South Africa in Section 6.)

Because acute episodes occur in most serious mental disorders the law should contemplate **emergency procedures**. These should allow the compulsory evaluation of persons with mental disorders and/or admission for 48-72 hours to allow assessment by a mental health specialist if there is a reasonable suspicion of an immediate risk to their health or safety.

Emergency procedures should be set out in law.

The law should also include provisions regarding the rights of individuals who are deprived of their liberty. All patients admitted involuntarily should have a specific right to appeal against their involuntary hospitalization both to the managers of the institution concerned and to a review board or tribunal (United Nations, 1991).

Patients should have the right to appeal against involuntary admission.

3.1.5 Voluntary and involuntary treatment in hospital settings

Voluntary treatment is associated with the issue of informed consent. The legislation must ensure that all treatments are provided on the basis of free and informed consent except in rare circumstances. Consent cannot be lawful if it is accompanied by a threat or an implied threat of compulsion or if appropriate alternatives to the proposed treatment are not offered for consideration.

Patients who are admitted voluntarily should only be treated after informed consent has been obtained. In the case of involuntary patients, important issues arise when procedures are being considered for both involuntary admission and involuntary treatment.

Several issues arise when procedures are being considered for both involuntary admission and involuntary treatment.

It is sometimes argued that the purpose of involuntary admission should be to provide treatment, i.e. to reverse deterioration in a person's condition, and that a failure to achieve this renders admittance purposeless and tantamount to incarceration. Two separate procedures, the first for involuntary admission and the second for administering involuntary treatment, could act as a barrier to treatment or delay it. In particular, developing countries with limited resources may have difficulties in performing separate examinations for admission and treatment.

It has also been argued that the task-specific and time-specific nature of competence means that patients who are not competent to decide about their admission may nevertheless be competent to give consent to treatment and make decisions on their treatment plans. In such cases, the argument runs, it is crucial that a person's competence to give consent to treatment is determined *before* any decisions on treatment are made.

The issue of separate procedures versus a single procedure for involuntary admission and involuntary treatment remains controversial. It is beyond the scope of this module to advocate the adoption of one approach rather than the other. It is necessary for each country to decide which is suitable. However, it remains essential that, in either case, sufficient safeguards are put in place to protect patients' rights and prevent abuses of the procedures.

If it is found that a patient lacks the capacity to give consent, involuntary treatment should be considered only if (1) the patient is admitted involuntarily to hospital **and** (2) the treatment is necessary to bring about an improvement in the patient's condition and/or restore her or his competence to make decisions about treatment and/or to prevent significant deterioration in the patient's mental health and/or to prevent self-harm or harm to other people.

There are specific criteria for involuntary treatment.

In the case of involuntary treatment, procedures should be established to protect the human rights of the person concerned and to provide protection from possible harm and misuse of the powers being used. The mechanisms may include obtaining a second opinion on the need for involuntary treatment, obtaining independent permission from judicial sources and/or patients' representatives, and appeal by the patient against involuntary treatment to an independent review body.

For certain treatments, legislation makes it compulsory to obtain informed consent. In addition a second opinion and permission from an independent judicial or quasi-judicial body is required for treatment to proceed. Many of these treatment modalities are controversial and their mention here should not be taken to imply endorsement by WHO. The primary concern is to acknowledge and emphasize the need for sufficient protection of the rights of people with mental disorders in given circumstances. Examples include psychosurgery, the implantation of medications to reduce sex drive, and seclusion procedures. These safeguards are generally applied to treatments which are considered irreversible and/or carry a relatively high risk of physical or mental harm for the patient.

3.1.6 Involuntary treatment in community settings

There is a growing demand for the supervision of persons with mental disorders in the community. This arises from both public and professional perceptions that deinstitutionalization has failed and that persons with mental disorders in the community pose a public risk (Harrison 1995; Thomas, 1995). Professionals have been concerned with the situation in which persons with mental disorders undergo involuntary admission and treatment, stop taking medication on being discharged, and then relapse, with the result that another cycle of involuntary admission and treatment is required.

Countries that have enacted legislation for community supervision orders (also called community treatment orders) usually require persons with mental disorders to reside at a specified place, to attend specified treatment programmes that include counselling, education and training, to allow mental health professionals to have access to their homes, and to submit to compulsory (involuntary) psychiatric treatment. (See, for example, the United Kingdom's Mental Health (Patients in the Community) Act 1995.

A concern with community supervision and treatment orders is that mental health services may come to rely on compulsion in the provision of community-based care, rather than focusing on making such services acceptable to people with mental disorders and investing effort and resources in engaging them in the services. This could undermine an important aim of deinstitutionalization.

An important issue concerning community supervision is that of consent to treatment. Persons residing in the community who have recovered from mental disorders have the competence and capacity to make decisions about their treatment. The right to give consent is accompanied by the right to refuse it, and this right must be respected. To act otherwise would be to suggest that persons with mental disorders had the capacity to give consent but not the capacity to refuse treatment, thus violating the principle of symmetry. The key point is that rules for involuntary treatment must be followed, i.e. a lack of capacity and a likelihood of danger to self or others has to be demonstrated.

The evidence base for the effectiveness of compulsory community supervision is only starting to be developed. Supervision orders appear to decrease re-hospitalization and total hospital-days when they are accompanied by intensive community-based treatment. This requires a substantial commitment of human and financial resources (Swartz et al., 1999). Sizeable reductions in the risk of violent behaviour is possible only if compulsory supervision is accompanied by intensive outpatient treatment

(Swanson et al., 1999). Such reductions are mainly attributable to an increase in adherence to treatment and a decline in the misuse of substances (Swanson et al., 1999).

The above is not a comprehensive review of the effectiveness of compulsory community supervision. However, it is clear that community supervision can work only if intensive community-based treatment facilities are available.

3.1.7 Periodic review mechanism

The legislation should provide for an automatic periodic review mechanism in all instances affecting the integrity or liberty of persons with mental disorders (United Nations, 1991). Thus there should be legislative provision for automatic review mechanisms in all cases of involuntary admission and treatment and in cases of voluntary admission and treatment that continues for more than a certain period. Reviews should take place at reasonable intervals, e.g. no longer than monthly for compulsory procedures and three-monthly for voluntary stays. They should be conducted by an independent regulatory body with legal or quasi-legal status for the enforcement good practice.

A review body is a monitoring mechanism ensuring the implementation of safeguards contained in legislation.

To be effective the reviewing body should:

a) be multidisciplinary and include professionals
   (mental health, legal, social work), representatives of people with mental
   disorders, representatives of their families, advocates and lay persons;
b) be financially and operationally independent of service providers
   and entities mandated to purchase services for persons
   with mental disorders;
c) have statutory powers to enforce compliance with the provisions
   of mental health legislation.

3.1.8 Competence (capacity)

For consent to be valid the person giving it must have the capacity to do so. Competence to give consent or refuse treatment refers commonly to the capacity to understand the purpose, nature, likely effects and risks of a particular treatment, including the likelihood of its success, the consequences of withholding it and any alternatives to it.

Capacity is a prerequisite for valid consent.

Mental disorders can affect competence. Legislation should therefore provide protection to people suffering from mental disorders. The presence of mental disorder does not automatically imply incapacity to make competent decisions. The law should lay down explicit procedures for assessing competence, should stipulate the appropriate authorities to determine competence, and should outline the actions to be performed if a person is deemed incompetent.

Mental disorder does not automatically imply incapacity.

In most jurisdictions, decisions on competence are made by the judicial authorities on the basis of the expert opinions of mental health professionals. Legislation in many countries contains provisions for the formal appointment of guardians for persons who are lacking competence because of mental disorders. There should be provisions in the legislation for appeal against incompetent decisions by affected individuals and/or their carers and families.

3.1.9 Accreditation for professionals and mental health facilities

Accreditation ensures satisfactory quality and uniformity in the provision of mental health services. (See *Quality Improvement for Mental Health*.) Users should have the satisfaction of knowing that minimum criteria for professional skills and quality of care have been met by both professionals and facilities. Legislation can provide for the setting up of accreditation systems and ensure that only accredited mental health facilities and professionals are allowed to provide services.

3.1.10 Rights and roles of families and carers

Families play an important role in supporting and caring for persons with mental disorders. This is especially so in countries lacking well developed state social security systems. The legislation should take account of the needs and rights of families and should balance them with the needs and rights of individuals with mental disorders. For example, families caring for relatives with mental disorders may require information from professionals about the nature of the illnesses and the current treatment plans so that they can care for their relatives effectively. The legislation should therefore deal with the need of families to gain access to such information when necessary. It should also ensure that individuals' needs for confidentiality are balanced against families' needs for information.

It is important to balance the needs and rights of families and carers with the needs and rights of individuals with mental disorders.

3.2 Substantive provisions for other legislation impacting on mental health

Legislation in areas outside the mental health sector can play an important role in the integration of persons with mental disorders into communities. Such legislative measures can help to ensure the success of a policy that promotes community-based care for mental disorders and deinstitutionalization. Legislation in these areas is also important in the prevention of mental disorders and the promotion of mental health.

3.2.1 Housing

Legislation can incorporate provisions for giving persons with mental disorders priority in state housing and in subsidized housing schemes, and can mandate local authorities to establish a range of housing facilities such as halfway homes and long-stay supported homes. Housing legislation should include provisions for preventing the geographical segregation of persons with mental disorders. This requires specific provisions for preventing discrimination in the siting, location and allocation of housing for persons with mental disorders.

Legislation can help to improve access to affordable housing of good quality.

3.2.2 Education

Children, youth and adults have the right to appropriate educational opportunities and facilities. Countries should ensure that the education of people with mental disorders is an integral part of the educational system. If necessary, curricula should be flexible enough to allow for additions or adaptations in order to accommodate the special needs of persons with mental disorders. Integrated education and community-based programmes should be seen as complementary approaches in providing cost-effective education and training for people with mental disorders.

The education of people with mental disorders should be an integral part of the education system.

Specific school mental health programmes have a role to play in the early identification of emotional and behavioural problems in children and thus in helping to prevent future disabilities caused by mental disorders. School-based programmes also help to increase awareness about emotional and behavioural disorders and to develop skills for coping with adversity and the management of stress.

3.2.3 Employment

Legislation can include provisions for the protection of persons with mental disorders from discrimination and exploitation in employment. This should include provisions for equal employment opportunities and for prohibiting employers from using mental disorder as a ground for removal from employment. There should be provisions for establishing

Legislation can help to prevent discrimination and the exploitation of persons with mental disorders in the workplace.

adequate funding of vocational rehabilitation programmes, for preferentially financing income-generating activities by people with mental disorders who reside in the community, and for general affirmative action programmes aimed at improving access to paid employment. Employment legislation can also provide protection for persons with mental disorders who are engaged in sheltered work schemes, ensuring that they are remunerated at rates comparable to those received by other people and that there is no forced or coercive labour in such schemes.

Employment legislation that incorporates a provision for maternity leave, especially paid maternity leave, has proved effective in many countries. It allows new mothers to spend more time with their infants at home and fosters bonding. Similar measures for fathers are being implemented in some developed countries.

Maternity leave promotes mental health in mothers and children.

3.2.4 Social security

Disability benefits are required for persons with mental disorders at similar rates to those granted to people with physical disabilities. The social security system should be flexible enough to allow people to obtain paid employment without losing their disability pensions.

Benefits for people with mental disabilities should be given at the same rate as those for people with physical disabilities.

3.2.5 Criminal justice

A country's criminal code should include provisions relating to offenders with mental disorders. These provisions should, for instance, deal with the competence of such offenders to stand trial and to act as witnesses in criminal proceedings, and with criminal responsibility, legal representation, sentencing and treatment (Bowden, 1995).

3.2.6 Civil and general purpose legislation

Persons with mental disorders are entitled to exercise all civil, political, economic, social and cultural rights as recognized in the Universal Declaration of Human Rights, the International Covenant on Economic, Social and Cultural Rights, and the International Covenant on Civil and Political Rights.

Legislation can protect the right of persons with mental disorders to exerc all their civil, political, economic and social righ

Provisions relating to marriage, separation, divorce and parental rights of persons with mental disorders can be incorporated into civil legislation. Alternatively, mental health legislation should state that persons with mental disorders have the following rights, among others:

- to vote
  (unless considered incompetent to do so);
- to marry;
- to have children
  and maintain parental rights;
- to own property;
- to employment;
- to education;
- to freedom of movement
  and choice of residence.

General purpose legislation can be made applicable to people with mental disorders by including them in it as beneficiaries. This is true, for example, of antidiscrimination legislation and affirmative action legislation for the protection of vulnerable populations, minorities and underprivileged groups.

3.2.7 General health care legislation

Persons with mental disorders need legislative protection in their interaction with the general health care system. The matters that have to be covered include access to treatment, the quality of treatment offered, confidentiality, consent to treatment and access to information. Special clauses can be inserted to emphasize the need to protect vulnerable people, e.g. those with mental disorders and those lacking the capacity to make decisions for themselves.

The low priority given to mental health issues in most countries results in mental health services receiving inadequate financial and human resources. In order to promote fairness and equity, therefore, general health care legislation should also include provisions for adequate resources and funding for mental health services both in institutional settings and in the community. This would result in the same level of access and quality of care for people with mental disorders as for those with physical disorders.

There should be equity in access to treatment of good quality as between persons with mental disorders and those with physical disorders.

In many countries, people need health insurance in order to obtain access to health care. General health care legislation in such countries should contain provisions for preventing discrimination against people with mental disorders in respect of obtaining adequate health insurance from public and private providers for the care and treatment of physical and mental disorders. Countries can formulate legislation that provides for the introduction of mental health interventions into primary care. For instance, early intervention, including the availability of essential psychiatric drugs, should be included in any basic health plan for the purposes of reimbursement or coverage of services (World Health Organization, 1996c).

Countries can formulate legislation that provides for the introduction of mental health interventions in primary care.

3.2.8 Access to psychotropic medications

Psychotropic drugs are useful for treating mental disorders and play an important role in secondary prevention. However, it is common for even basic psychotropic drugs to be unavailable in many countries. Legislative action can help to improve the availability of drugs at the primary and secondary care levels.

Legislation can help to improve the availability of psychotropic drugs.

3.2.9 Protection of vulnerable groups

Protection of children and adolescents, women and elderly people. Many countries and international organizations have recognized the deleterious effect of physical abuse, sexual abuse, exploitation and labour on the mental health of children and adolescents. These issues should be considered an important component of mental health legislation. For example, legislation can be developed that ensures early detection of child abuse by health professionals and prompt communication to the judicial system (World Health Organization, 1996b). Similarly, it is often necessary for legislation to overcome gender inequalities for women in health, education and employment and to recognize physical and sexual abuse as criminal offences (World Health Organization, 1997a). The protection of the rights of elderly people is another component that should be considered in mental health legislation (World Health Organization, 1997b).

The legislation should protect vulnerable groups.

Protection of indigenous ethnic groups and minorities. Indigenous ethnic groups and minorities are among the most vulnerable groups of people, with high rates of depression, alcoholism, suicide and violence. They have experienced rapid cultural change, marginalization and absorption into a global economy that has little regard for their autonomy. Their level of mental health can be raised by means of laws that reinforce their identity, community life, local control and cultural traditions. They also require mental health services that accord with their cultures and languages and, ideally, that incorporate traditional forms of healing (Kirmayer, 2000).

3.2.10 Restricting access to alcohol and drugs

Legislation restricting physical access to alcohol and drugs can make a significant contribution to the prevention of abuse and dependence. In the case of alcohol, such measures include the enactment of a minimum legal drinking age, restrictions on the hours and days of sale, and restrictions on the numbers and locations of retail outlets (Edwards, 1997).

Legislation that restricts access to alcohol and drugs can prevent abuse and dependence.

Key points: Vital components of mental health legislation

- The legislation should not only protect the rights of people with mental disorders but should also aim to promote mental health and prevent mental disorders.

- The legislation should embrace the principle of the least restrictive alternative, requiring that people are always offered treatment in settings that will least restrict their personal freedom and least affect their status and privileges in the community, allowing them to continue to work, move about and deal with their affairs.

- The legislation should guarantee the confidentiality of all information on people with mental disorders which is obtained in a clinical context.

- The principle of free and informed consent to treatment should be enshrined in the legislation.

- Involuntary admission to hospital should only occur exceptionally and in very specific circumstances. The legislation should outline these exceptional circumstances and lay down the procedures to be followed for involuntary admission.

- Involuntary treatment should only be considered in certain rare situations, e.g. if they lack the capacity to consent and the treatment is necessary to improve their mental health condition and/or prevent a significant deterioration in their mental health and/or prevent injury or harm to themselves or other people.

- In countries where there is involuntary treatment in the community, the rules for such treatment should be established and followed, i.e. a lack of capacity and a likelihood of danger to self or others should be demonstrated.

- The legislation should contain a provision for the appointment of an independent review body to act as a regulatory mechanism with specified composition, powers and duties.

- Legislation should not be restricted to issues of mental health or even general health. Legislation on housing, education, employment and general health, among other matters, is also important for the promotion of mental health and the prevention of mental disorders and should therefore receive adequate attention.

4. The drafting process: key issues and actions

This step begins once the political will exists for incorporating the components discussed in the previous section into national legislation. The task of drafting the legislation is best performed by a specially constituted committee, the composition of which is important. It should represent a sufficient diversity of expertise to reflect competing ideologies. The participation of users and carers is crucially important but frequently neglected.

The drafting committee should include:

- one or two persons representing the ministry of health, usually including the professional in charge of mental health, who can chair the committee or act as its executive secretary;
- one or two persons from the other ministries involved;
- legislators with an interest in mental health;
- representatives of people with mental disorders, carers and advocacy organizations;
- mental health professionals;
- lawyers with expertise in mental health and other sectors;
- experts with experience of working with women, children and the elderly.

The drafting committee should be representative of diverse opinions.

Consultation should start before drafting begins and should continue until the implementation stage. The initiation of dialogue before the process begins enables the identification of key and controversial issues at an early stage and can promote action, enthusiasm and a desire for change among stakeholders.

Once the legislation has been drafted it should be presented for consultation to all the key stakeholders in the mental health field. If it is well planned and systematically executed, consultation can have a positive impact on the adoption of the proposed legislation and its implementation. Consultation also provides an opportunity to raise public awareness about several issues. These include the needs of persons with mental disorders, the prevention of mental health problems, community involvement and the increased visibility of mental disorders. In this way the likelihood is increased of effective implementation of the legislation once it has been enacted.

The consultation process can have a positive impact on the implementation of legislation.

Further advantages of the consultation process include the identification of potential weaknesses in the proposed legislation, of potential conflicts with existing legislation and local customary practices, and of issues inadvertently omitted from the draft legislation, and the raising of possible practical difficulties of implementation.

Consultation should follow a time-limited three-stage process that includes:

- the publication of the draft document in the print and electronic media of the country concerned and an invitation to the general public to respond;
- inviting written responses from the public, organizations and representatives of the relevant government authorities and nongovernmental agencies;
- regional and national public meetings conducted by the drafting committee to analyse, discuss and negotiate the most frequent and important objections or suggestions made in connection with the drafted legislation.

Box 4. Key stakeholders who should be invited for consultation about proposed mental health legislation

- Government agencies, including the ministries of health, finance, justice, education, employment (labour) and social welfare

- Politicians, legislators and opinion-makers

- Law enforcement agencies such as the police and the prison service

- Judicial services

- Representatives or associations of families and carers of persons with mental disorders, advocacy organizations representing the interests of such persons, and user groups

- Academic institutions and professional bodies representing professionals such as psychiatrists, psychologists, psychiatric nurses and medical and psychiatric social workers

- Profit as well as not-for-profit nongovernmental agencies providing care, treatment and rehabilitative services to persons with mental disorders

- Religious authorities

- Other special interest groups such as minority organizations and groups representing tribal minorities

At the end of the consultation phase it is useful for the drafting committee to publish a report on suggestions, objections and queries received during the consultation process and the committee's response to them. Sections of the proposed legislation which have received substantive objections, especially from user groups and advocacy organizations, should be given particular attention. It is advisable for the committee to give a detailed response to any substantive objections that it does not accept and that, in the opinion of the committee, do not require any modifications, alterations or changes to the proposed legislation.

Key points: The drafting process

- The drafting committee should comprise a sufficient diversity of expertise to reflect competing ideologies.

- The participation of people with mental disorders and carers is crucially important in the drafting process but is frequently neglected.

- The draft legislation should be presented for public consultation.

- Consultation provides an opportunity to raise awareness about mental disorders and to identify potential weaknesses in the proposed legislation, areas inadvertently omitted and difficulties of implementation.

- Consultation should be time-limited and should involve all the important stakeholders.

- At the end of the consultation phase the drafting committee should publish a report on it which includes the suggestions put forward and the changes made to the draft legislation.

5. Adoption of legislation: key issues and actions

Mobilizing public opinion crucial for the adoption of legislation.

This is potentially the most time-consuming step. Progress with the proposed legislation can easily be slowed down by technicalities at this stage. It is necessary to persuade politicians and key members of the executive branch of government and the legislature about the urgent need for new mental health legislation and consequently for adequate legislative time to be made available. Although government support will have been given for the formation of the drafting committee, once a final document is ready to be sent to the legislature, there may be other political issues at stake. Especially in low-income countries, mental health has a low political priority and competes for time and resources with many other pressing problems.

Support from public opinion can be used to persuade decision-makers. Efforts to gain public support should begin as early as possible, preferably during the consultation process. As mentioned in Section 4, expert consultation provides an opportunity to raise public awareness about the topics included in the proposed legislation. This should continue during the present step. Media strategies can be useful and the professionals in charge of mental health in the ministry of health should provide journalists with material for news, reports and interviews. Workshops and seminars can be held for key groups and organizations so that the main components of the new legislation can be explained and discussed. It is also useful to enlist the support of individuals who already have high visibility, are credible and have a positive image. These people can act as spokespersons to deliver the message about mental health and the need for legislation.

Mental health advocacy groups can play a valuable role in these activities. The process of adopting and implementing new legislation presents an opportunity to empower these organizations in their fight against the marginalization and stigmatization of people with mental disorders. Thus a mental health law that aims to achieve a normal life within the community for persons with mental disorders could well become a vehicle for educating people, influencing social attitudes and facilitating social change. (See *Advocacy for Mental Health*.)

Lobbying members of the executive branch of government and the legislature is another important activity for stimulating the adoption of proposed mental health legislation. The members of the legislature should be informed of the deficiencies in the existing legislation on mental health or of the negative consequences of the absence of such legislation. It is necessary for them to understand the social need for the proposed law, the principal ideas on which the draft is based, the probability that the future law will solve existing problems, and other relevant issues.

Lobbying plays an important role in promoting the adoption of legislation

The persons in charge of mental health in the ministry of health should conduct frequent meetings with key members of these institutions as well as with politicians from the whole spectrum of political parties. Periodically, these people should receive documents that contain information on mental health and best practice and that invite them to give their opinions about policy and legislative initiatives. Lobbying is essential throughout the legislative process, particularly during adoption, in order to ensure that the proposed law is sent to the legislature and that it advances through the stages of analysis, discussion and promulgation.

Some of the obstacles and solutions to formulating and adopting mental health legislation are indicated below.

Obstacles and solutions to formulating mental health legislation

Obstacles	Solutions
Tension between people in favour of mental health legislation on treatment and patient' rights and those in favour of legislation on promotion and prevention.	Appoint a drafting committee with representatives from both groups to enable frank and open discussion between the parties and to ensure that both perspectives are included in the draft legislation.
Power struggle between doctors and lawyers making it difficult to reach consensus.	Formulate a mental health law from the perspective of people with mental disorders and include a participative process with many sectors and disciplines.
Tension between the rights and responsibilities of families and the rights and responsibilities of people with mental disorders.	Organize workshops involving members of both groups to analyse human rights and family roles.
Resistance from psychiatrists to a decrease in their independence to indicate treatments, including those given on an involuntary basis.	Hold seminars on the rights of people with mental disorders and medical ethics, with the participation of international experts.
Low priority given to mental health legislation by government, parliament and sectors outside health.	Empower organizations of consumers, carers and other advocacy groups. Lobby legislators and find individual legislators who may be prepared to promote mental health legislation.

Key points: adoption of legislation

- The adoption of legislation may be delayed because of other legislative priorities, especially in developing countries.

- Mobilizing public opinion and lobbying legislators can hasten the adoption of legislation.

6. Implementation: obstacles and solutions

It is preferable for the process of implementation to begin from the point of conception of mental health legislation. Many implementation difficulties can be identified and corrective action can be taken during the drafting and consultation phase of proposed legislation. The complexity of modern mental health legislation adds to the difficulties of practical application. Much attention is frequently paid to the drafting and legislative process while little preparatory work is done on implementation until after the legislation has been enacted. The early identification of issues can help with the implementation process. Experience gained in many countries shows that "law in books" and "law in practice" are sometimes rather different. It is entirely understandable that there should be problems of implementation in relation to newly adopted legislation in countries lacking a tradition of mental health law. However, problems of this kind also occur in countries with a history of such legislation.

Many countries have mental health legislation that is not adequately implemented.

6.1 Obstacles

Difficulties with implementation may arise for several reasons.

6.1.1 Lack of coordinated action

User groups, family groups and advocacy organizations in developed countries act as catalysts for implementation, occasionally using the judicial process in this connection. The relative scarcity of such groups in developing countries leads to slower implementation through gradual change in customary practices. This problem is compounded by the fragmentation of the groups that do exist and a lack of coordinated action. Consequently, many of the potential benefits of mental health legislation are never passed on to persons with mental disorders.

6.1.2 Lack of awareness

The general public, professionals, people with mental disorders, their families and advocacy organizations are frequently ill-informed about the changes brought about by new mental health legislation. In some instances they may be well informed about these changes but remain unconvinced about the reasons for them. This is especially true if mental health legislation requires significant changes in customary practices.

6.1.3 Human resources

In developing countries there are acute shortages of appropriately trained mental health professionals. For example, mental health legislation usually requires that a statement be obtained from a psychiatrist before involuntary admission to hospital takes place. This may be a significant obstacle to implementation in developing countries because psychiatrists may only be available in urban areas whereas the vast majority of people live in rural areas.

6.1.4 Procedural issues

Little attention is paid to operationalizing legal concepts into practical procedures and standardizing documentation for compliance with the provisions of mental health legislation. These deficiencies lead to patchy implementation or, occasionally, a complete failure to implement legislation. For example, it is helpful for clinicians and others if there is a standardized proforma for certification, and users and their families are likely to find it useful to have a standard proforma for appeals against admission.

6.1.5 Lack of finances

The speed and quality of implementing legislation is likely to depend on the availability of adequate financial resources. New mental health legislation usually requires a shift from institutional to community-based care and this requires additional funding. In the long run, the reallocation of funds from institutions to community-based facilities is feasible. In the short-term, however, there is a need to meet double running costs during the transition phase.

In countries lacking a publicly funded health care system, opposition may come from providers of mental health care who complain of increased costs attributable to the implementation of mental health legislation. In such countries the families of people suffering from mental disorders bear the financial burden and consequently they too are likely to complain of increased costs arising from legislative changes.

6.2 Strategies for overcoming implementation difficulties

The following suggestions may help to overcome implementation difficulties.

6.2.1 Finances

Adequate budgetary provision is essential for activities that are intended to achieve speedy implementation. For example, funds are required for setting up the activities of a review body, training mental health professionals in the use of legislation, and effecting changes in mental health services. In most cases, these budgetary provisions are included in the general health care budget. However, the low priority given to mental health may result in budgets intended for mental health being diverted to other areas of health care. In such instances, it is therefore important to ensure that budgets for mental health care are protected and utilized only for their intended purpose. (See *Mental Health Financing*.)

6.2.2 Coordination

A coordinating authority or agency should be created to oversee the implementation of mental health legislation. This body should have a timetable, measurable targets, and administrative and financial powers enabling it to ensure effective and speedy implementation. It should have the mandate, authority and adequate financial resources to:

- develop rules and procedures for implementation;
- prepare standardized documentation instruments;
- ensure a proper process for training mental health professionals
  and introducing certification procedures if necessary;
- address human resource issues, e.g. by empowering adequately trained
  and supervised non-medical mental health professionals (nurses, nursing
  aides, psychologists, psychiatric social workers) to act as specialists
  in certain situations.

Developing countries may find it difficult to create a coordinating agency because of a lack of human resources. In some countries this role can be assumed by the people in charge of mental health policy and planning in ministries of health, with help from review bodies (Section 3.1.7) and advocacy organizations.

6.2.3 Wide dissemination among people with mental disorders, families and advocacy organizations

The provisions of new legislation should be disseminated among important stakeholders such as groups representing people with mental disorders, families of such people and advocacy organizations by means of workshops and seminars. Groups representing people with mental disorders are being established and increasing their level of activities in many developing countries, e.g. Brazil, Mexico, and Uganda. (See Advocacy for Mental Health.) It is important that these groups be seen as partners in the implementation of new mental health legislation and that they be included in implementation strategies.

6.2.4 Public education and awareness

A public education and awareness campaign should be targeted at the general public, highlighting the substantial provisions of the new legislation and, in particular, the rationale and philosophy underlying the changes.

6.2.5 Training for general health, mental health and other professionals

A knowledge of mental health legislation is extremely important for its proper implementation. It is therefore necessary to promote special training for general health and mental health professionals and staff, law enforcement officers, lawyers, social workers, teachers, human resource administrators, and so on. Training courses for mixed groups of general health and mental health professionals and other professionals outside the health sector may lead to a better understanding of mental health and mental disorders and of the human rights of persons with mental disorders, and may help to establish a common language between professionals in different disciplines.

6.2.6 Visiting boards for mental health facilities and procedures for complaints and redress

Regular monitoring visits to mental health facilities provide a valuable safeguard against unjustified involuntary detention and the limitation of patients' rights. The people entrusted with implementing legislation should ensure that the review body speedily sets up boards of visitors for mental health facilities. In addition, there should be rapid and effective implementation of complaints procedures as provided in the legislation. Such mechanisms are supplementary to other general procedures for appeals against administrative decisions that violate civil and human rights.

Key points: Implementation

- Many countries have mental health legislation that is not adequately implemented.

- Implementation difficulties can be identified and corrective action can be taken during the drafting and consultation phase of proposed legislation.

- Such difficulties may arise because of a lack of coordinated action for implementation, a lack of awareness, a paucity of human resources, procedural issues and a lack of finances.

- A coordinating agency with a clear timetable and measurable targets can facilitate the implementation process.

- Additional funds are required for implementation and there should be adequate budgetary support to facilitate it.

- User groups, families, carers and their organizations and advocacy organizations are useful partners in connection with hastening the process of implementing new legislation.

- A public campaign can increase awareness about new legislation and thus directly and indirectly influence its implementation.

7. Recommendations and conclusions

This section lists recommendations for the professionals or teams responsible for mental health in ministries of health. The recommendations are intended to facilitate the development of national mental health legislation. Countries in the initial phase of the legislative process which have no mental health legislation (7.1) or a limited amount of such legislation (7.2) should find the subsequent recommendations (7.3 and 7.4) useful at a later stage in the drafting, adoption and implementation processes.

7.1 Recommendations for countries with no mental health legislation

1. Set priorities for mental health legislation in accordance with the realities of the country concerned.
2. Review health and non-health legislation in the country in order to identify places where priority mental health components can be incorporated.
3. Obtain support for mental health legislation from the main stakeholders in the country and try to achieve a preliminary agreement with them about the content of the legislation and the strategy to follow in implementation.
4. Lobby key members of the executive branch of government, ministries, legislature and political parties in order to obtain an officially appointed drafting committee.
5. If you do not obtain immediate support from these people, empower organizations of consumers, carers and other advocacy groups, and organize with them a public education and awareness campaign to highlight the need and rationale for mental health legislation. (See *Advocacy for Mental Health*.)

7.2 Recommendations for countries with a limited amount of mental health legislation

1. Map the existing mental health legislation of the country in question in order to show its components exactly.
2. Set priorities for new components of mental health legislation with reference to what is missing and to modifications required in existing legislation.
3. If there is no specific mental health legislation in the country, consult with the main stakeholders in order to establish the pros and cons of having such legislation. Decisions have to be taken in accordance with the cultural, social and political situation in the country. The most effective approach is likely to involve a combination of specific mental health legislation and components integrated into existing laws.
4. Lobby key members of the executive branch of government, ministries, legislature and political parties in order to obtain an officially appointed drafting committee.
5. If you do not obtain immediate support from these people, mobilize and empower organizations of consumers, carers and other advocacy groups, and organize with them a public education and awareness campaign in order to highlight the need and rationale for new mental health legislation (See *Advocacy for Mental Health*.)

7.3 Recommendations for countries with drafted mental health legislation that has not been adopted

1. Lobby key members of the executive branch of government, ministries, legislature and political parties with a view to the drafted legislation being sent to the legislature and moved forward through the different steps (commissions and plenary sessions).
2. If the drafted documents do not move forward, mobilize and empower organizations of consumers, carers and other advocacy groups, and organize with them a public education and awareness campaign in order to highlight the need and rationale for new mental health legislation. (See *Advocacy for Mental Health*.)
3. If the progress of the drafted document continues to be held up, review it with the drafting committee in order to identify stumbling blocks or areas of resistance and try to address these through further debate and discussion.

7.4 Recommendations for countries with mental health legislation that has not been adequately implemented

1. Map the mental health laws of the country in question and set priorities for the components that are in most urgent need of implementation.
2. Conduct interviews with key informants and/or focus groups involving people with mental disorders, carers, mental health professionals and other stakeholders in order to identify the main barriers to the adequate implementation of mental health legislation.
3. If one of the barriers is resistance by the population because of misinterpretation or a lack of information, conduct a public education and awareness campaign to highlight the rationale for and provisions of mental health legislation. (See *Advocacy for Mental Health*.)
4. If there is a shortage of mental health staff or resistance from professional groups, conduct training programmes for key professional groups.
5. If there is insufficient funding to develop the mechanisms needed to implement the law (e.g. advocacy, awareness, training, visiting boards, complaints procedures), establish partnerships with key stakeholders. (See *Advocacy for Mental Health*.)

8. Country examples of mental health legislation

> In most rural areas and many poorer urban areas of **South Africa** there are very few psychiatrists or medical practitioners with knowledge and experience of psychiatry. However, there are a number of highly skilled and experienced nurses who do have a knowledge and experience of psychiatric practice. Furthermore, there are other health professionals, e.g. psychologists and occupational therapists, who are able to conduct mental health assessments. The former legislation stated that two medical practitioners, one of them a psychiatrist, were required to do an initial examination for the certification of persons with mental disorders. New legislation has introduced the category of the mental health care practitioner. The skills required of such practitioners are not written into the legislative document but are prescribed by regulation. Thus flexibility is built into the legislation: as the number of mental health professionals increases the criteria for acceptance as a mental health care practitioner can be narrowed down by modifying the regulations. Through this process the country has been able to build legislation around the realities of its human resources.

> WHO has provided technical cooperation in connection with the formulation of the Mental Health Law in the **Republic of Korea** since 1982. International experts visited the country and workshops were organized. Korean psychiatrists and administrators started to draft of a mental health law based on a Japanese law of 1987. The Ministry of Health and Social Affairs submitted the final draft to the National Parliament in October 1993. WHO representatives were asked to visit the Republic of Korea in March 1994 to review the draft of the Mental Health Law, which was approved by Parliament in the same year. The law gives families an important role, allowing compulsory admission of persons with mental disorders to hospitals on the basis of the agreement of family members and certified psychiatrists. This contrasts with what happens in Western countries, where individual free will is strongly protected.

> **Italian** Public Law 180, enacted in 1978, and the Mental Health Act of 1983 in **England and Wales**, are radical examples of a shift from custody and incarceration to the integration and rehabilitation of persons with mental disorders. In both instances, the emphasis is on the voluntary treatment of persons with mental disorders in the community and integrated health institutions, as opposed to segregated mental asylums. Patients can thus integrate into community life. Admissions to psychiatric wards in hospitals are not predicated on a perception that patients are dangerous but on an urgent need for forms of treatment that can only be provided if patients stay in hospital.

> In the **Russian Federation** a law on psychiatric care was passed in 1992. It placed some emphasis on protecting the human rights of people with mental disorders, but did not question the established conceptual and organizational basis of care provision.

> The 1999 **Belarusian Mental Health Law** contains important statements concerning the human rights of persons with mental disorders and has provisions for preventing the abuse of authority by professionals and others. It also regulates involuntary admissions to hospital and the discharge of patients in emergency cases. The procedures of admission and discharge and their judiciary aspects accord with generally recognized international law.

> In **Japan** the Mental Hygiene Law was enacted in 1950. It encouraged the development of psychiatric hospitals and ensured financial support for patients who were admitted involuntarily. This resulted in very long stays in hospital, the building of several private psychiatric hospitals and a dramatic increase in the number of psychiatric beds to 360 000 (29 per 10 000 population). These figures were among the highest in the world.

Concerns were expressed about the violation of the human rights of persons admitted to these hospitals. A new Mental Health Law was passed in 1987, stressing the importance of the human rights of inpatients and supporting the development of community-based mental health services. In 1993 the Basic Welfare Law for the Disabled was passed and in 1994 the Community Health Care Law was enacted. In 1995 the Mental Health Law of 1987 was reformulated as the Mental Health and Welfare Law, promoting the development of integrated medical and welfare services for people with mental disorders.

> A patients' advocacy service with broad functions has been introduced in **Austria**. It provides legal representation for patients committed by the courts to psychiatric hospitals. It delivers counselling and information on patients' rights for patients, their families and friends, and other interested people. Two non-profit associations run the service. They are responsible for training, guiding and supervising patients' advocates and, in turn, are supervised by the Austrian Federal Ministry of Justice. The services of patients' advocates are confidential and free of charge to patients. Every involuntary patient is entitled to the services of such an advocate.

> In the **Province of Rio Negro, Argentina**, a mental health law was enacted in 1991 which consolidated a profound transformation of psychiatric services into community and general hospital care which had begun in 1985. Between 1991 and 1993 the number of professionals and staff working in community mental health teams increased by approximately 50%. The participation of members of families, friends and community volunteers in therapeutic activities, as stated in the law, increased dramatically, and the numbers of mental health professionals and staff working in general hospitals increased by 25% (Cohen, 1995).

> **Pakistan** recently enacted new mental health legislation in the form of Mental Health Ordinance 2001, which replaced the Lunacy Act of 1912. The new legislation emphasizes the promotion of mental health and the prevention of mental disorders and encourages community care. It is hoped that it will help to establish national standards for the care and treatment of patients and that it will help to promote public understanding of mental health issues.

> In **Trinidad and Tobago**, legislation appropriate to the time was enacted in 1975. The country adopted a new mental health plan in March 2000. Subsequently the Government appointed a committee chaired by the Manager of Legal Services in the Ministry of Health to draft a new mental health law. The committee has produced draft legislation that is currently circulating among key stakeholders for comment. After this phase the draft legislation will be forwarded to Cabinet, which will then decide on a time frame for inclusion on the legislative agenda.

> **Tunisia** promulgated a law regulating mental health care in 1992. The following conditions have to be fulfilled if involuntary admission and treatment of persons in mental health facilities are to take place: a) the persons suffer from mental disorders necessitating immediate care; b) the persons are unable to give informed consent; c) the persons pose a risk to their own safety or that of other people. Decisions are made and reviewed by a judicial authority and are based on the recommendations of two doctors, at least one of whom is a psychiatrist. Involuntary admission is limited to three months initially. Persons who are admitted involuntarily have the right to appeal against such decisions.

The same law contains sections guaranteeing persons with mental disorders the right to exercise all their civil, economic and cultural rights unless they are placed in the care of a guardian. A review board chaired by a judge and including psychiatrists and representatives of local authorities is entrusted with the task of periodically reviewing the cases of all persons who are admitted involuntarily to mental health facilities. The board is also expected to conduct regular inspections of all mental health facilities.

A broad range of other laws helps to promote mental health and prevent mental disorders. Thus:

(1) psychiatry has recently been added to the list of medical priorities,
giving financial incentives to encourage specialists to settle in the country;
(2) drug consumption has been prohibited since 1956 but a recent amendment
has allowed for the treatment of substance abuse and dependence
and has led to the opening of a substance use treatment centre;
(3) the rehabilitation of persons with mental disorders is facilitated
by a law that reserves 1% of all jobs in businesses with 100
or more employees for persons with disabilities;
(4) mental health care is guaranteed to prisoners;
(5) legislation ensures the rights of the child;
(6) legislation promotes gender equality through provisions relating
to the institution of legal divorce, recognition of the right of spouses of both
genders to seek divorce, the setting of a minimum age for marriage for women,
compulsory education for all boys and girls, and the maintenance
of equal opportunities in employment.

> In **China** the drafting process has lasted more than 16 years. The current draft, which is the thirteenth version, has sections on: the protection of civil rights, including employment and education rights, of persons with mental disorders; informed consent; confidentiality; voluntary and involuntary hospitalization and treatment; rehabilitation and community-based mental health services; the promotion of mental health; and the prevention of mental disorders. Many stakeholders consider mental health legislation as being concerned with only care, treatment and the provision of institution-based services. There is resistance to change from professionals and the established health system. Many professionals fear that the enactment of new legislation will increase the probability of their being blamed by patients and relatives for failures of the system. Consequently, professionals such as psychiatrists and nurses, potentially the most enthusiastic proponents of new legislation, remain indifferent to the issue. Since 1998 there have been efforts to speed up the process of adopting mental health legislation. Activities undertaken during 2002 included survey and research work identifying the country's principal mental health problems and barriers, studies on the components of legislation in countries socially and culturally similar to China, and efforts to build a consensus for change (Dr Xie Bin, personal communication, 2002).

Capacity / Refers more specifically to the presence of the physical, emotional and cognitive abilities to make decisions or to engage in a course of action.

Competence / Refers more specifically to the legal consequences of not having capacity. There are commentators, however, who define capacity as the ability to make an informed choice with respect to a specific decision, and use competence to mean the ability to process and understand information and to make well-circumscribed decisions on that basis.

Consolidated mental health legislation / All issues of relevance to persons with mental disorders, viz. mental health, general health and non-health areas are included in a single legislative document.

Discrimination / Arbitrary denial of rights to persons with mental disorders, that are afforded to other citizens. Laws do not actively discriminate against people with mental disorders but can place improper or unnecessary barriers or burdens on them.

Dispersed mental health legislation / A strategy of inserting provisions relating to mental disorders into legislation related to particular areas. The legislation is applicable to all persons, including those with mental disorders.

Regulations / A set of rules that are not part of legislation but are based on certain principles outlined in it. The procedure for framing such regulations is outlined in the legislation.

References

1.   Arjonilla S, Parada IM, Pelcastre B (2000) Cuando la salud mental se convierte en una prioridad. [When mental health becomes a priority]. *Salud Mental*, 23(5):35-40. In Spanish.

2.   Bowden P (1995) Psychiatry and criminal proceedings. In: Chiswick D, Cope R, eds. *Seminars in practical forensic psychiatry*. London: Royal College of Psychiatrists.

3.   Cohen H, Natella G (1995) *Trabjar en salud mental, la desmanicomialización en Rio Negro [Working on mental health, the deinstitutionalization in Rio Negro]*. Buenos Aires: Lugar Editorial. In Spanish.

4.   *Community psychiatry in Italy*. Giordano Invernizzi, http://www.pol-it.org

5.   Council of Europe (1994) *Council of Europe Parliamentary Assembly Recommendation 1235 on Psychiatry and Human Rights*. Council of Europe.

6.   Pan American Health Organization/World Health Organization (1990) *Declaration of Caracas, adopted at the Regional Conference on the Restructuring of Psychiatric Care in Latin America*, Convened in Caracas, Venezuela. PAHO/WHO.

7.   World Psychiatric Association (1996) *Madrid Declaration on Ethical Standards for Psychiatric Practice*. World Psychiatric Association. http://www.wpanet.org

8. Edwards G, et al. (1997) *Alcohol policy and the public good.*
Oxford: Oxford University Press.

9. Harrison K (1995) Patients in the community. *New Law Journal* 276:145.

10. Jegede RO, Williams AO, Sijuwola AO (1985) Recent developments in the care,
treatment and rehabilitation of the chronic mentally ill in Nigeria.
Hospital and Community Psychiatry 36:658-61.

11. Kirmayer LJ, Brass GM, Tait CL (2000) The mental health
of aboriginal peoples: Transformations of identity and community.
Canadian Journal of Psychiatry 45:607-16.

12. Swanson JW, et al. (2000) Involuntary outpatient commitment
and reduction in violent behaviour in persons with severe mental illness.
British Journal of Psychiatry 176:324-31.

13. Swartz MS, et al. (1999) Can involuntary outpatient commitment reduce hospital
recidivism? Findings from a randomised trial with severely mentally ill individuals.
American Journal of Psychiatry 156:1968-75.

14. Thomas T (1995) Supervision registers for mentally disordered people.
New Law Journal 145:565.

15. United Nations (1991) *Principles for the Protection of Persons with Mental
Illness and for the Improvement of Mental Health Care (Resolution 46/119).*
New York: United Nations General Assembly.

16. United Nations (1993) *The Standard Rules on the Equalization of Opportunities
for Persons with Disabilities, United Nations General Assembly, Resolution 48/96.*
New York: United Nations General Assembly.

17. United Nations (1966) *International Covenant on Civil and Political Rights
(Resolution 2200A (XXI).* New York: United Nations General Assembly.

18. United Nations (1966) *International Covenant on Economic,
Social and Cultural Rights, United Nations General Assembly Resolution 2200A (XXI).*
New York: United Nations General Assembly.

19. Wachenfeld M (1992) The human rights of the mentally ill in Europe under the
European Convention on Human Rights. *Nordic Journal of International Law* 107:292.

20. World Health Organization (1996a) *Guidelines for the promotion of human
rights of persons with mental disorders.* Geneva: World Health Organization.

21. World Health Organization (1996b) *Mental health care law: ten basic principles.*
Geneva: World Health Organization.

22. World Health Organization (1996c) *Global action for the improvement
of mental health care: policies and strategies.* Geneva: World Health Organization.

23. World Health Organization (1997a) *A focus on women.*
Geneva: World Health Organization.

24. World Health Organization (1997b) *Organization of care in psychiatry of
the elderly: a technical consensus statement.* Geneva: World Health Organization.

25. World Health Organization (2001) *Atlas: Mental health resources in the world, 2001*. Geneva: World Health Organization, Department of Mental Health and Substance Dependence.